Soft Tissue Sarcoma and Leiomyoma - Diagnosis, Management, and New Perspectives

Edited by Gamal Abdul Hamid

Published in London, United Kingdom

Soft Tissue Sarcoma and Leiomyoma - Diagnosis, Management, and New Perspectives
http://dx.doi.org/10.5772/intechopen.110954
Edited by Gamal Abdul Hamid

Contributors
Ahmed R. Eldesoky, Aliyu I. Lawan, Antarip Bhattacharya, Asmaa A. Abdeltawab, Demetrio Larraín, Eseoghene Dase, Jaime Prado, Minakshi Vashist, Mohamed Kelany, Noha Mohamed, Olakunle A. Azeez, Priya Sharma, Reetu Hooda, Rohit Kaushik, Shadrach M. Pius, Sonia Narwal, Sunita Singh, Supratim Bhattacharyya, Usman R. Yahaya, Vandana Kalra, Vinay V., Yves-Marie Robin

First published in London, United Kingdom, 2024 by IntechOpen
IntechOpen is the global imprint of INTECHOPEN LIMITED, registered in England and Wales, registration number: 11086078, 167-169 Great Portland Street, London, W1W 5PF, United Kingdom

British Library Cataloguing-in-Publication Data
A catalogue record for this book is available from the British Library

Additional hard and PDF copies can be obtained from orders@intechopen.com

Soft Tissue Sarcoma and Leiomyoma - Diagnosis, Management, and New Perspectives
Edited by Gamal Abdul Hamid
p. cm.
Print ISBN 978-0-85466-356-9
Online ISBN 978-0-85466-355-2
eBook (PDF) ISBN 978-0-85466-357-6

Meet the editor

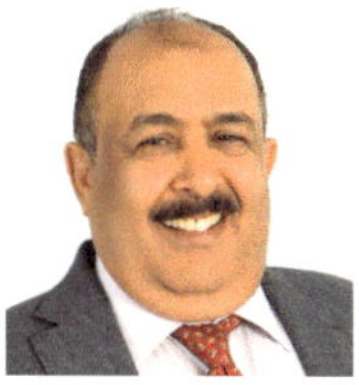

Prof. Dr. Med Gamal Abdul Hamid received his board certification in internal medicine and Ph.D. in Hematology-Oncology from the Faculty of Medicine (Caral Gustav Carus), University of Dresden, Germany. Currently, he is the general director of a national program of cancer control and professor of hematology-oncology at the University of Aden, Yemen. He is the general secretary of the Yemen Cancer Society and founder of the Aden Cancer Registry. He is an editorial member and reviewer of several hematology-oncology journals. He has also authored and co-authored numerous journal articles and delivered lectures at many conferences and institutions in Yemen and internationally. He is a member of the European Society for Medical Oncology, the American Society of Clinical Oncology, The International Network for Cancer Treatment and Research, Panarab Oncology, and The World Academy of Medical Sciences.

Contents

Preface

Soft tissue tumors are one of the difficult areas of oncological diagnosis. Diagnostic pathology results from a complex series of morphological observations, molecular genetics, cytogenetics, and immunohistochemistry. This book focuses on benign, moderate, and malignant soft tissue tumors that underlie the major diagnostic pitfalls. It discusses the differential diagnosis, classification, pathogenesis, and treatment of uterine fibroids, uterine leiomyomas, and emerging mesenchymal tumors.

It addresses the clinical and molecular diagnosis of soft tissue sarcomas and the classification and histopathology of the tumor as the basis for treatment recommendations, including surgery, radiation, and systemic therapy. This book provides specific chemotherapy and targeted treatment and immunotherapy for each sarcoma subtype, as well as presents a practical, modern approach to treating the many subtypes of soft tissue sarcomas.

The book is organized into two sections: "Soft Tissue Sarcoma – Diagnosis and Management" and "Uterine Leiomyoma – Diagnosis and Management". The chapters synthesize an enormous amount of scientific and clinical data and provide a comprehensive overview to create state-of-the-art descriptions of soft tissue sarcoma and leiomyoma.

This book, a collaboration of experts in the field, is an important resource for surgeons, oncologists, pathologists, epidemiologists, and postgraduate students who diagnose, treat, and research all known soft tissue tumors and hereditary tumor syndromes. It conveys the intricacy of soft tissue tumors as well as the variety of approaches to their diagnosis and treatment.

Dr. Gamal Abdul Hamid
Professor,
Faculty of Medicine,
University of Aden,
Aden, Yemen

Section 1

Soft Tissue Sarcoma – Diagnosis and Management

Chapter 1

Management of Soft Tissue Sarcoma

Mohamed Kelany, Ahmed R. Eldesoky, Asmaa A. Abdeltawab and Noha Mohamed

Abstract

Soft tissue sarcomas are a diverse category of rare malignant tumors that originate from mesenchymal tissues, such as muscles, nerves, and adipose tissues. They exhibit substantial morbidity and mortality due to the frequent development of advanced and metastatic conditions. Several challenges have been reported in diagnosis and treatment, with a shift toward molecular characterization and subtyping. Targeted therapy for certain forms of soft tissue sarcomas has seen significant advancements in the previous two decades. Many novel therapeutic strategies have been developed and approved as a result of the ability to study these molecular markers linked to the genesis of sarcomas. An overview of soft tissue sarcoma diagnosis and treatment is given in this chapter.

Keywords: soft tissue sarcoma, limb-sparing surgery, tyrosine kinase inhibitors, rare cancers, retroperitoneal sarcoma

1. Introduction

Sarcomas are a rare heterogeneous group of malignancies that originated from connective tissues in any organ or at any anatomic location of the body [1]. Their name originates from the Greek term for a fleshy excrescence. In his book Surgical Observations, published in 1816, the Edinburgh surgeon Charles Bell (1772–1842) introduced the term soft tissue cancer. According to the literature, he was the first to use the term soft tissue sarcoma to differentiate it from carcinoma. Despite the diversity of different types of tissues and locations, these soft tissue sarcomas (STS) are grouped because of their overall similarities in natural history and treatment ([2], pp. 1803–21).

Sarcoma accounts for fewer than 1% of all adult cancers and 10% of pediatric tumors. In the US, about 11,000 new cases are diagnosed annually, which accounts for less than 1% of total cancer cases. Approximately 80% of sarcoma originates from soft tissue, and the rest originates from bone. Most sarcomas (about 55%) affect mainly the extremities, mostly the legs, and about 15% affect the head and neck area or trunk; the rest are retroperitoneal or intraperitoneal [3].

With an estimated 27,908 new cases annually in the EU27, the overall crude incidence was 5.6 per 100,000 per year. Of these, 84% were soft tissue sarcomas and 14% were bone sarcomas [4].

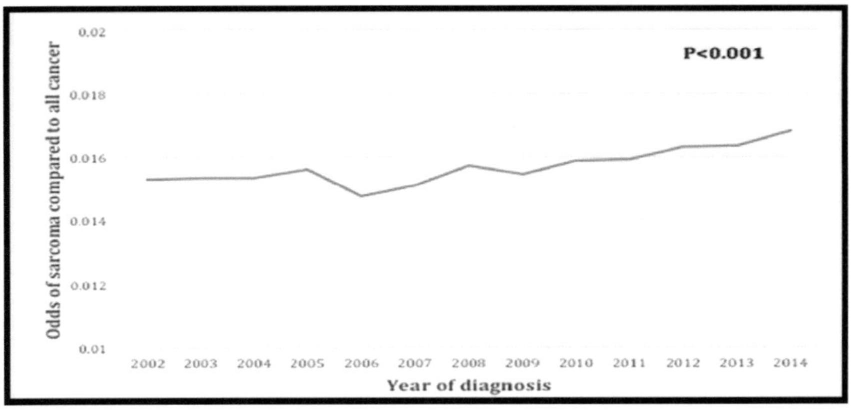

Figure 1.
Trends in the UK's sarcoma incidence over time [5].

The overall incidence of soft tissue sarcoma has increased in the UK over time due to improvements in diagnostic techniques and accurate recording within the cancer registries. It is interesting that over the last decades (between 1999 and 2001 and 2008–2010), incidence rates have increased by 17% in males but have not changed significantly in females (**Figure 1**) [6].

There are different reasons for these dynamic changes regarding the incidence: one reason is the histopathological reclassification and change of subtype definition; for example, atypical lipomatous tumors have been included in the category of well-differentiated liposarcoma, and therefore liposarcoma incidence rates began to rise. In contrast, gastrointestinal stromal tumors (GISTs) were classified separately from leiomyosarcoma, and consequently, leiomyosarcoma incidence rates began to fall [7]. The second reason is changes in reporting practice using accurate diagnostic tools, which allow more specific coding by cancer registries. A third reason is a change in the etiological factors, for example, the incidence of angiosarcoma of the breast is increasing due to the growing number of women receiving radiotherapy for breast cancer [6].

Rhabdomyosarcoma is most frequently diagnosed in pediatric patients, whereas synovial sarcoma, Ewing sarcoma, osteosarcoma, desmoplastic small round-cell tumors, clear cell sarcoma, alveolar soft part sarcoma, epithelioid sarcomas, and malignant peripheral nerve sheath tumors are more frequently diagnosed in adolescents and young adults [8].

Among adult sarcoma patients, undifferentiated sarcomas, gastrointestinal stromal tumors, leiomyosarcomas, and liposarcomas are the most frequent cancers [9].

Research investigating gender disparities has revealed that males have a greater prevalence of STS in comparison to females. According to Hung et al., it was observed that there was a notable prevalence of males among the 11,393 patients with soft tissue sarcomas (STS) [10].

2. Risk factors

2.1 Genetic redeposition

The development of bone and soft tissue sarcoma has been associated with several inherited genetic disorders, particularly in children and young people [11].

Li-Fraumeni syndrome (LFS) is distinguished by genetic alterations in the TP53 gene. Also, TP53 is the most prevalent germline mutation that predisposes to pediatric sarcomas, including osteosarcoma, undifferentiated pleomorphic sarcoma, rhabdomyosarcoma, leiomyosarcoma, and liposarcoma. The prevalence of LFS in children with soft tissue sarcomas is estimated to be 7% [12]. Among a specific cohort of persons in the International Agency for Research on Cancer (IARC) database, 96% of the sarcomas that developed in individuals with LFS occurred before the age of 50. This is in contrast to the general population, where only 38% of sarcomas occur before the age of 50 [13].

Familial adenomatous polyposis (FAP) is a genetic condition caused by a mutation in the APC gene located at 5q21-q22. Familial adenomatous polyposis (FAP) patients often experience intra-abdominal desmoid fibromatosis, which is also called desmoid tumors. This combination is also known as Gardner syndrome [14].

The retinoblastoma RB1 gene is associated with soft tissue sarcoma, particularly leiomyosarcoma [15].

Double hit inactivation, a condition in which one allele is activated in the germline and the second allele is eliminated by somatic mutation, is the source of mutations in the NF1 gene that results in neurofibromatosis type 1, an autosomal dominant illness. This disease is diagnosed by major criteria, including café-au-lait spots, neurofibroma, plexiform neurofibroma, iris nodules, and bone deformity, as well as other factors [16]. Up to 13% will develop soft tissue sarcoma, mostly in the form of malignant peripheral nerve sheath tumors [17].

2.2 Molecular alternation in sarcomas

The conventional karyotypic analysis derives much of the current molecular understanding of sarcomas [18]. At the cytogenetic level, it discriminated sarcomas into two main categories: sarcomas with a simple karyotype versus those with a complex karyotype. From a biological perspective, there is a greater level of comprehension regarding the oncogenic pathways associated with sarcomas that possess a simple karyotype. These mechanisms may generally be classified into two overarching categories: transcriptional deregulation and unregulated signaling. In contrast to sarcomas characterized by highly complicated karyotypes, which generally lack singular "driver" genetic mutations, sarcomas with nonspecific molecular changes are more prevalent. These changes contribute to the development of oncogenic features, including dysregulation of the cell cycle and genomic instability (**Figure 2**) [19, 20].

2.3 Environmental factors

2.3.1 Radiation exposure

Murray et al. [5] revised and updated the original radiation-associated sarcoma (RAS) diagnosis criteria in 1999 to include all varieties of radiation-associated sarcoma. Murray et al. outlined the following requirements: First, the patient must have a historical context that involves the occurrence of sarcoma in the region encompassed by the radiation field and the 5% isodose line. Additionally, it is crucial to establish the absence of any indications of sarcoma prior to the administration of radiation therapy. Furthermore, the sarcomas must be confirmed through histological evidence and exhibit distinct pathological characteristics in

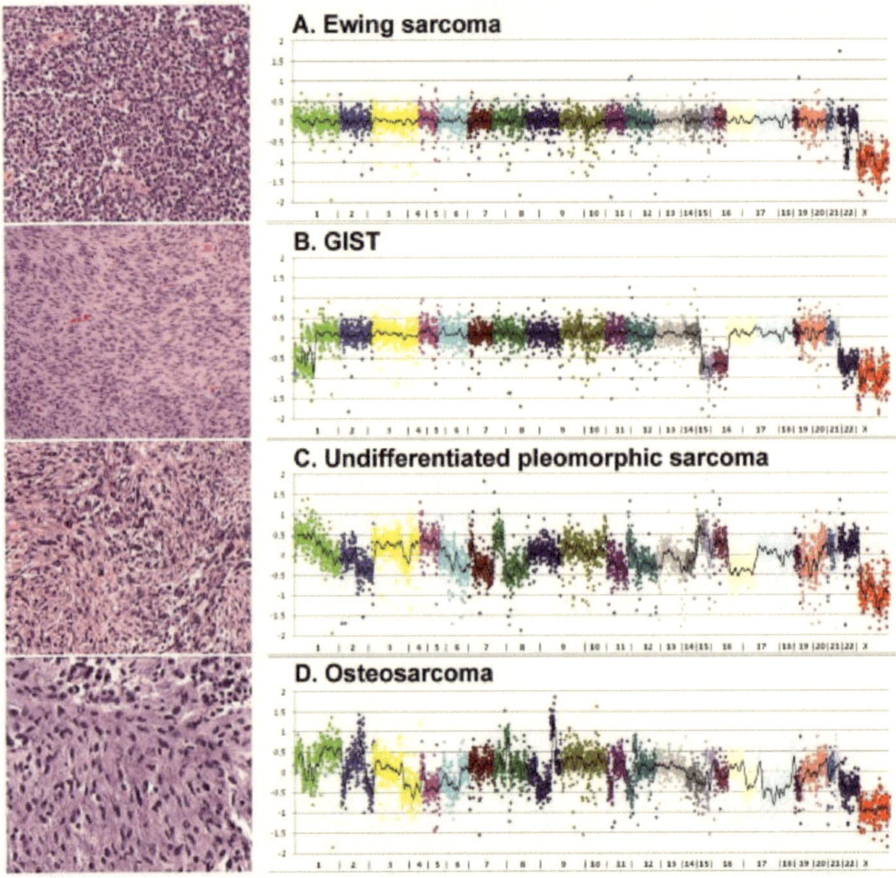

Figure 2.
The copy number patterns of sarcomas characterized by a simple genome (top) and sarcomas characterized by a complex genome (bottom), as determined using a next-generation sequencing platform. The case under consideration involves a 9-year-old male patient who has been diagnosed with Ewing sarcoma. The genetic profile is characterized by its simplicity. The presence of an EWSR1-FLI1 fusion was detected in this tumor using the aforementioned assay. The patient in question is a 60-year-old male who has been diagnosed with a high-risk, spindle cell intestinal gastrointestinal stromal tumor (GIST). The presence of a KIT K642E mutation was identified in the tumor using the test. The observed genomic profile exhibits a very straightforward genetic makeup, featuring a nearly diploid karyotype and the absence of chromosomes 1p, 14q, 15q, and 22q. These chromosomal losses are indicative of advanced gastrointestinal stromal tumors (GIST). C. Undifferentiated pleomorphic sarcoma originating in the deltoid muscle of a 55-year-old male individual, and the case under consideration involves a 7-year-old male patient diagnosed with conventional osteosarcoma in the femur. The genetic analysis of this condition reveals the presence of several chromosomal gains and losses, which occur in a nonrecurrent manner. Both tumors had genetic changes in the TP53 gene, namely including copy number loss and truncating mutations [19].

comparison to the primary tumor. The latency period for the onset of radiation-induced sarcoma generally ranges from 5 to 20 years [21].

An examination of 20 instances of radiation-induced sarcoma, which includes four instances that were treated using carbon ion radiotherapy, the histological diagnoses of RAS included leiomyosarcoma, undifferentiated pleomorphic sarcoma, rhabdomyosarcoma, angiosarcoma, malignant peripheral nerve sheath tumor, and spindle cell sarcoma, not otherwise specified [22].

2.3.2 Chemical exposure

Sarcoma development has been linked to several substances. However, it is challenging to identify obvious causal effects due to the limited patient numbers in cohorts. Hepatic angiosarcoma has been linked to the chemical vinyl chloride, which was used in the plastics industry in the 1970s [23].

A review of 31 studies and 29,605 cancer cases found that higher levels of 2,3,7,8-tetrachlorodibenzo-p-dioxin were linked to the development of STS [24].

2.3.3 Trauma exposure

Numerous papers documenting the occurrence of secondary traumatic stress (STS) following traumatic injury, surgical procedures, and other related experiences [25–27] show that trauma exposure has a causal relationship with the development of STS. However, establishing a causal relationship between the two occurrences is a significant hurdle. This phenomenon can be attributed, in part, to the tendency of trauma to bring attention to a preexisting mass located in the same area.

2.4 Infectious and immunological factors

Despite the role of infectious agents in the development of sarcoma is not well understood, there is strong evidence for the association between viral infection and sarcoma development. HIV infection and human herpes virus 8 are known as causative factors for Kaposi sarcoma. Also, leiomyosarcoma has been connected to Epstein-Barr virus infections in patients with HIV infection [28].

In addition, it has been suggested that the acquired regional immune deficiency in combination with chronic lymphedema after exposure to radiation therapy or an infectious condition may lead to the development of angiosarcoma [29].

3. Diagnosis and staging

3.1 Anatomical imaging of soft tissue sarcoma

3.1.1 Ultrasound (US)

It is used to confirm the existence of a soft-tissue mass and determine its size, depth, and consistency to guide core-biopsy sampling of superficial masses [30].

Accuracy improved the distinguishing between the aggressive and benign lesions in the US based on echotexture, in which the large, deep-seeded lesion with internal heterogeneity and mass effect raised suspicion of neoplasia. In addition, the vasculature and the high-grade neoplasm were associated with increased peripheral flow because of neoangiogenic and central avascular areas due to necrosis [25].

3.1.2 Computed tomography (CT)

CT is the most accurate modality for evaluating osseous architecture. In soft tissue sarcoma, CT is a very helpful method for the detection of cortical bone invasion, periosteal reaction, and dystrophic calcification seen in some synovial sarcoma.

Furthermore, CT angiography readily demonstrates the vascular anatomy [26].

3.1.3 Magnetic resonance imaging (MRI)

The most sensitive and accurate imaging technique for assessing soft-tissue masses. It provides the finest delineation of the soft-tissue structures and the relation of the mass to neurovascular structures. Thus, it is the study of choice for the localization and staging of soft-tissue tumors [27].

In magnetic resonance (MR) imaging, commonly employed sequences encompass regular T1 and T2-weighted pictures. The incorporation of fluid-sensitive and fat-saturated sequences serves to enhance specificity. It is worth noting that the MR signal intensity characteristics exhibited by most soft tissue lesions, such as soft tissue sarcomas, and lack specificity. The observed tendency is for moderate signal intensity to be displayed on T1-weighted pictures in comparison to skeletal muscle, whereas high-signal intensity is displayed on T2-weighted images [26].

When considering different subtypes of soft tissue sarcoma, some characteristics observed in magnetic resonance imaging (MRI) scans can potentially indicate the specific subtype of sarcoma. The high amount of myxoid matrix in myxofibrosarcoma has been linked to a higher chance of local recurrence after surgery (see **Figure 3**). The "tail sign" and "water-like" appearance on fluid-sensitive sequences are signs of this. In cases of undifferentiated pleomorphic sarcoma, the presence of the "tail sign" is also linked to a higher chance of local recurrence after surgery [31, 32].

The presence of the "triple sign" in magnetic resonance imaging (T2w sequences) of synovial sarcoma patients is linked to reduced disease-free survival. This sign indicates the concurrent existence of solid cellular elements (with intermediate signal intensity), hemorrhage or necrosis (with high signal intensity), and fibrotic regions (with low signal intensity) [31].

3.2 Functional and molecular imaging

The glucose-transporter family (GLUT) found in cellular membranes is one commonly used method for tumor imaging. This family of transporters plays a crucial role in regulating the intake of glucose. Tumors exhibit overexpression of the most significant subtypes, namely GLUT 1 and GLUT 3. Tumor cells exhibit a higher demand

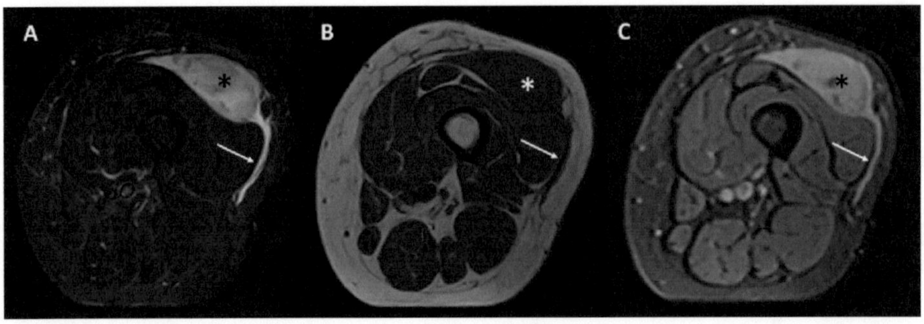

Figure 3.
Contrast-enhanced MRI scans in a 61-year-old woman with myxofibrosarcoma of the left thigh A, precontract axial short inversion time inversion recovery scan, and B, precontract axial T1-weighted scan, show a neoplastic lesion located above the fascial plane with two components—A main mass (*) and a so-called tail sign (arrow), both with the same signal intensity. C after contrast, an axial T1-weighted scan with fat saturation shows that both the main mass (*) and the tail sign (arrow) have a lot more contrast [31].

for glucose to support their proliferation, which can be attributed to the inefficient process of aerobic glycolysis, also known as the Warburg effect [33].

It has been found that the metabolic features of 18F-FDG PET/CT are strongly linked to the histological grade of soft tissue sarcomas (STS). According to sources [34, 35]. For instance, the utilization of both visual and quantitative analysis of FDG PET images could facilitate the distinction between liposarcomas and lipomas. The average standardized uptake value (SUV) of myxoid-type lipomas and other types of liposarcoma was statistically significantly higher than that of a well-differentiated liposarcoma by two and three times, respectively [36, 37].

The use of whole-body FDG PET-CT has demonstrated its ability to serve as a supplementary tool in the process of staging and restaging many types of malignancies, including STSs. The study results demonstrated that the rates of sensitivity and specificity in detecting lung metastases using FDG PET were 86.7 and 100%, respectively. By contrast, the CT scan by itself exhibited sensitivity and specificity rates of 100 and 96.4%, respectively. In comparison, the CT scan alone had sensitivity and specificity rates of 100 and 96.4%, respectively [38]. The user's text does not contain any information to rewrite. In addition, the FDG PET-CT scan revealed the presence of 13 additional sites of metastases that were not anticipated. More research has shown that positron emission tomography-computed tomography (PET-CT) can find more lymph nodes and bone lesions when first evaluating a soft tissue sarcoma (STS) compared to using only traditional imaging methods. Nevertheless, it exhibited reduced sensitivity and specificity in detecting pulmonary metastases [39, 40].

3.3 Biopsy

The current recommendation for the detection of soft tissue sarcomas (STS) is percutaneous core needle biopsy (CNB), sometimes referred to as "tru-cut biopsy." This approach is preferred due to its minimally invasive nature and its ability to preserve the option for future surgical procedures without limitations. The accuracy of this procedure is comparable to that of an incisional biopsy, while offering the advantage of not needing hospitalization [41].

In the most extensive cohort of individuals, core needle biopsy (CNB) demonstrated a sensitivity of 99.4% and a specificity of 98.7% when utilized for the purpose of distinguishing between malignancy (specifically sarcoma) and benign mesenchymal tumors [14]. The observed percentages closely resemble those obtained by utilizing the incisional biopsy technique. Similarly, CNB can accurately determine the histological subtype and grade in 80% of instances [42].

An inappropriate biopsy may lead to excess bleeding with a chance of spreading sarcoma cells by hematoma beyond the original site. Inexpert surgery may lead to the opening of tissue planes permitting further contamination of hematoma, which creates an even greater dilemma if contaminated hematoma involves vital anatomic structures such as nerves, vessels, and joints, for which sacrifice may result in significant functional consequences such as altered limb function or even amputation [43].

For this reason, all biopsies should be undertaken at a center specializing in sarcoma management. At these centers, there will be resources to ensure that the tissue is handled appropriately and expeditiously between the time of biopsy and histological examination. When the biopsy is taken outside of a specialized center, it is advisable that it occur after discussion with experts from a specialized sarcoma center [43].

Using radiological tools like ultrasonography and computed tomography (CT) to guide core needle biopsy (CNB) has greatly improved the effectiveness of diagnostic procedures. The utilization of image guidance facilitates enhanced precision in determining the location of tumors, hence assisting in directing biopsies toward regions containing live cancer cells. When determining the appropriate regions for biopsy, it is imperative to refrain from selecting cystic, necrotic, or hemorrhagic tumor regions. The meticulous evaluation of imaging studies is essential for identifying regions of heightened aggressiveness within tumors, typically characterized by a greater degree of contrast enhancement. This process enables a more precise determination of the cancer grade. The most often employed needle gauges for central neuraxial blocks (CNB) range from 14 to 18 g [44].

Prior to performing a percutaneous biopsy, it is imperative to address any hemostatic issues. Additionally, it is crucial to carefully select the biopsy site to avoid noninvolved anatomical compartments that may pose a risk of contaminating neurovascular structures. Furthermore, it is important to acknowledge that the biopsy path and resulting scar should be surgically resected in a definitive manner (**Figure 4**) [45, 46].

3.4 Soft tissue tumors pathology

The pathologist initially focuses on comprehending the clinical and radiological aspects of a soft tissue tumor. Understanding these characteristics, along with the

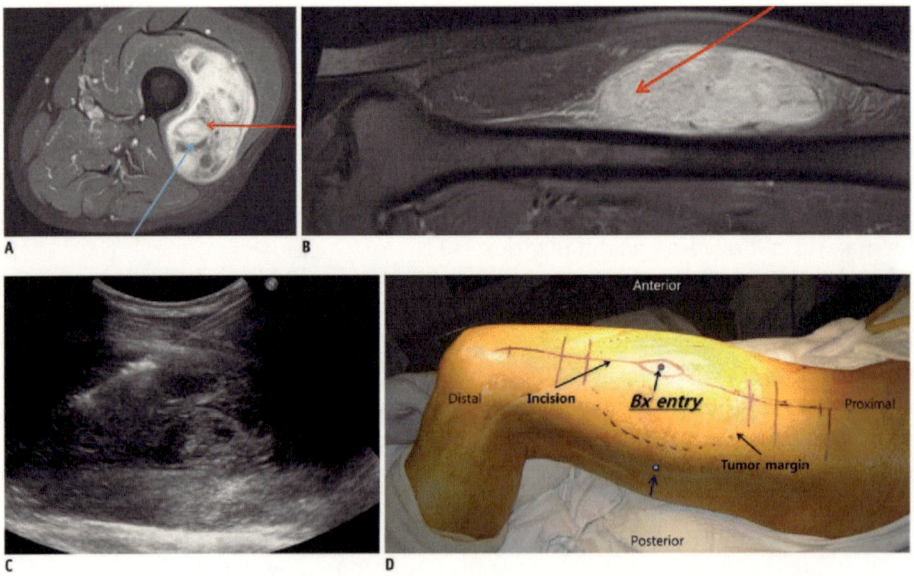

Figure 4.
(A), (B) Sagittal enhanced T1-weighted pictures, there is a solid mass present that exhibits heterogeneous enhancement. This mass affects the vastus intermedius and vastus lateralis muscles. The blue and red arrows represent two general potential pathways for performing a biopsy. The blue pathway traverses and interrupts the unaffected posterior compartment, but the red route exclusively passes through the anterior compartment, rendering it the suitable pathway. In this case, a longitudinal ultrasound (US) image was utilized to guide the core needle biopsy (CNB) procedure on the mass, following the red route. In the captured image of the left upper leg, it was observed that the biopsy entry site was situated appropriately within the designated surgical area and aligned with the intended incision line for the scheduled surgery. Blue markers (shown by a blue arrow) delineate the hypothetical path of a blue biopsy. The identification of this tumor has been verified as undifferentiated pleomorphic sarcoma [45].

Age	Soft tissue tumors
Infants (<3 years)	Infantile fibrosarcoma, inclusion body fibromatosis fibrous hamartoma of infancy lipoblastoma Myofibroma
Pediatric	Embryonal rhabdomyosarcoma, extrarenal rhabdoid tumor
Adolescence and young adults (<30 years)	Synovial sarcoma, alveolar rhabdomyosarcoma alveolar soft part sarcoma epithelioid sarcoma, epithelioid hemangioendothelioma, desmoplastic small round-cell tumor, low-grade fibromyxoid sarcoma, myxoid liposarcoma, inflammatory myofibroblast sarcoma, nodular fasciitis
Adults (<40 years)	Clear cell sarcoma, dermatofibrosarcoma protuberans, epithelioid hemangioendothelioma fibroma of tendon sheath, myositis ossificans
Adults (middle age)	Intramuscular myxoma, spindle cell lipoma Liposarcoma well-differentiated and dedifferentiated types, extra-skeletal myxoid chondrosarcoma, solitary fibrous tumor
Elderly/older adults	Atypical fibroxanthoma, myxofibrosarcoma Undifferentiated pleomorphic sarcoma

Table 1.
Summary of common soft tissue tumors based on the age of the patient [47].

evaluation of pathological findings, enables the consideration of potential alternative diagnoses. Relevant factors considered encompass the patient's age (**Table 1**), as well as the magnitude and location of the patient's condition. The following tables demonstrate the common tumors based on age and location.

Obtaining the patient's past medical history is crucial, as certain cancers may have connections or be linked to a syndrome, as explained in the genetic risk factor. Neurofibromatosis-1 (NF-1) is linked to the presence of neurofibromas and malignant peripheral nerve sheath tumors (MPNST) [17]. Familial adenomatous polyposis (FAP) is associated with intra-abdominal desmoid fibromatosis [14].

Finally, the diagnostic approach for soft tissue tumors is based on cellular morphology and immunohistochemistry (IHC), as well as molecular studies.

3.4.1 Cellular morphology

Spindle cell morphology is one of the most often observed histologic subtypes in soft tissue tumors. It is characterized by cells with thin, elongated nuclei and cytoplasmic borders with pointed or tapering ends.

Examples of spindle cells are smooth muscle tumors, nerve sheath tumors, nodular fasciitis, solitary fibrous tumors, synovial sarcoma, dermatofibrosarcoma protuberans, and fibromatosis. Given the vast and diverse differentials within the spindle cell group of tumors, other histological factors must be assessed to determine the correct diagnosis. This includes consideration of the architectural arrangement of the cells, the growth pattern, associated vascular pattern, background stroma or matrix, mitoses, and necrosis [48].

Epithelioid pattern: Epithelioid refers to cells that resemble epithelial cells in appearance and are spherical or polygonal with lots of cytoplasm. Soft tissue tumors that exhibit epithelioid cytomorphology are uncommon, either in their initial form (such as epithelioid sarcomas) or as the epithelioid variants of mesenchymal tumors, including leiomyosarcoma, fibrosarcoma, GIST, and vascular and neural tumors [48].

Round cell pattern: Small round blue cells are relatively uniform cells with a high nuclear-to-cytoplasmic ratio that appear dark blue on H&E stain. Tumors with round cells are more aggressive and frequently affect pediatrics. Immunohistochemistry is nearly always required for the diagnosis, and molecular methods are often used for gene fusions that characterize round-cell tumors [48].

Round-cell malignancies include both mesenchymal and non-mesenchymal tumors. Non-mesenchymal tumors include lymphoma, melanoma, and some carcinomas (Merkel cell and small cell carcinoma). Mesenchymal round-cell tumors include rhabdomyosarcoma, neuroblastoma, desmoplastic small round-cell tumor, poorly differentiated synovial sarcoma, Ewing's sarcoma, and undifferentiated round-cell sarcomas (previously called Ewing-like/atypical Ewing), CIC-rearranged sarcoma, and BCOR-rearranged sarcoma. Round cell areas can be seen in myxoid liposarcoma and mesenchymal chondrosarcoma. There is a major role for IHC and molecular typing in this category of tumors.

Myxoid pattern: myxoid tumors of the soft tissue are a broad, heterogeneous group of tumors that are characterized by their abundance of extracellular matrix. These tumors range from benign lesions, such as myxoma, angiomyxoma, and myoepithelioma, to malignant tumors, such as extra-skeletal myxoid chondrosarcoma, low-grade fibromyxoid sarcoma, and myxofibrosarcoma [43].

Adipocytic/lipomatous tumors: adipocytic tumors comprise a large group of heterogeneous tumors that display various pathological appearances and distinct clinical behaviors. These tumors can often present diagnostic challenges due to their overlapping features in histology. Benign fatty tumors include areas of fat necrosis, angiolipoma, hibernoma (brown fat), spindle cell lipoma, intramuscular lipoma, and lipoblastoma. Malignant liposarcoma has three main subtypes: WD/DD liposarcoma (**Figure 5**), myxoid liposarcoma, and pleomorphic liposarcoma [43].

Undifferentiated tumors: undifferentiated or unclassified tumors encompass a subset of tumors that display markedly atypical cells in the absence of any obvious line of differentiation on histology. A prominent example of these tumors is undifferentiated pleomorphic sarcoma (UPS), a highly aggressive tumor that accounts for 5–10% of all sarcomas arising in adults. Previously, UPS belonged to a larger entity

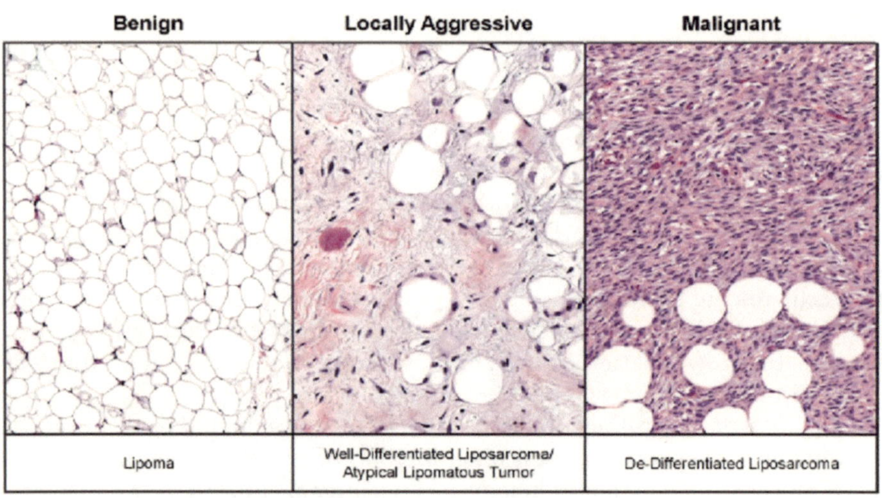

Figure 5.
Select tumors of adipocytic differentiation [43].

called malignant fibrous histiocytoma (MFH), a diagnosis previously given to poorly differentiated mesenchymal tumors that could not be otherwise classified [49]. With the addition of ancillary testing, it is now understood that MFH encompassed a heterogeneous group of both mesenchymal and non-mesenchymal tumors that shared similar histological features [50]. Nowadays, UPS is typically the diagnosis of exclusion for undifferentiated mesenchymal tumors, following immunohistochemical interrogation for other sarcoma entities [51].

3.4.2 Immunohistochemistry (IHC)

Immunoprofiles are not only useful in identifying the lineage of a tumor but also in supporting the diagnosis of rare tumors or tumors that have occurred in unusual situations or sites. The technique employs manufactured antibodies that bind to and identify the proteins (antigens) expressed by cells. The technical aspects of this method will influence its ability to detect an antigen in tumor tissue. Firstly, there needs to be enough representative tissue that is well-processed. Identifiable tumor tissue needs to be present in the sample.

In general, IHC can be used not only in the identification of the line of differentiation, summarized in **Table 2**, but also as a surrogate to identify specific molecular alterations. See **Table 3**.

3.4.3 Molecular testing

There are some chromosomal translocations found in histological subtypes that can be diagnosed by molecular techniques such as FISH and RT-PCR. See **Table 3**.

AJCC 8th edition	
T1	Tumor ≤5 cm in greatest dimension
T2	Tumor >5 cm and ≤ 10 cm in greatest dimension
T3	Tumor >10 cm and ≤ 15 cm in greatest dimension
T4	Tumor >15 cm in greatest dimension
N0	No regional lymph node metastasis or unknown lymph node status
N1	Regional lymph node metastasis
M0	No distant metastasis
Ml	Distant metastasis
Stage groups	
Stage IA	T1; N0; M0; G1
Stage IB	T2, T3, T4; N0; M0; G1
Stage II	T1; N0; M0; G2/3
Stage IIIA	T2; N0; M0; G2/3
Stage IIIB	T3, T4; N0; M0; G2/3
Stage IV	Any T; N1; M0; any G Any T; any N; M1; any G

Table 2.
Staging system for extremity soft tissue sarcoma or trunk [52, 53].

Epithelioid markers	Keratin cytokeratin Ck, pan ck, epithelial membrane antigen EMA	Positive in epithelioid sarcoma, synovial, desmoid round-cell tumor DRCT, epithelioid type leiomyosarcoma, rhabmyosarcoma, angiosarcoma
Myogenic markers	Desmin, SMA, myogenine, myod, HHF35 (muscle-specific antigen).	Desmin positive in smooth & skeletal muscles, DRCT, myofibroblast SMA, H- caldemin positive in leiomyosarcoma Myogenin myod positive in rhabdomyosarcoma
Endothelial markers	CD31, CD34, D2-40	CD34 positive in solitary fibrous tumor SFT, peripheral nerve sheath tumor PNST, dermatofibrosarcoma perturbance DFSP, epithelioid sarcoma, angiosarcoma. Cd31 positive in angiosarcoma, Kaposi, EHE. D2-40 highly specific in Kaposi sarcoma
Neural crest & melanoma markers	S100, Melan-A, HMB-45	S100 positive in schwannoma, neurofibroma, PNST, clear cell sarcoma, extra-skeletal myxoid chondrosarcoma, myoepithelioma. Melan-A positive in PECOMA.

Table 3.
IHC immunohistochemistry in the identification of line differentiation [43].

A prospective multicenter study (GENSARC) showed that molecular methods can modify diagnosis and thus affect management plans [54].

Molecular methods, such as fluorescence in situ hybridization (FISH) and reverse transcriptase polymerase chain reaction (RT-PCR) to find the protein products of these fusion genes, can help with the diagnosis of soft tissue sarcoma because several histologic subtypes are linked to particular chromosomal translocations [54].

3.5 Staging

The tumor, node, metastasis (TNM) approach was created in cooperation between the American Joint Committee on Cancer and the Union for International Cancer Control (UICC) and is the most popular staging method for soft tissue sarcomas (AJCC). The AJCC TNM system divides soft tissue sarcomas into stages based on tumor size (T), lymph node involvement (N), the presence or absence of distant metastases (M), and histologic grade (G) [52].

There are some updates, like the creation of different staging methods at various anatomical regions. It is well recognized that STSs that develop in the head and neck, retroperitoneum, or abdominopelvic cavities, or in the extremities or trunk (see **Table 2**), and show distinctions in their biological function and clinical outcomes [52].

4. Treatment of localized STS

Delivering treatment necessitates a multimodality team that consists of skilled pathologists, radiologists, orthopedic and reconstructive surgeons, radiation oncologists, medical oncologists, nurses, physical therapists, social workers, and radiation oncologists. The total removal of the tumor with the best possible function preservation and the least amount of side effects are the intended therapeutic outcomes. Due to the complexity of achieving these objectives, a skilled team in a specialized sarcoma center is best suited to handle STS treatment [55].

4.1 Surgery

4.1.1 Principles of surgery for extremity STS

Surgery with a negative margin is the standard primary treatment for most sarcomas. For surgical planning, local disease staging is crucial. Imaging of the affected site should include plain radiography, CT, MRI, or PET, as was previously stated. The precise position and approach to the mass must be carefully planned before proceeding with the biopsy. The following data are essential for designing the surgical margins and reconstructions: size, capsule, consistency, site, shape, edge, and nearby structures, as well as evaluating the response of neoadjuvant therapy [56].

Amputation: Primary amputation may occasionally be the only possible choice or may be required if a serious complication arises. Current indications for primary amputation for soft tissue sarcoma (STS) include massive disease, where a functional limb following resection is not achievable; the need for resection of certain major nerves (e.g., brachial plexus), vessels, and bone; or severely compromised tissue perfusion. Or on local recurrence with widespread lesions and no other options found [57].

The predominant reasons for amputation were patients presenting with either primary localized disease (33.3%) or recurrent disease (52.2%), where there was significant involvement of bone, muscles, and limb-sparing surgery was not feasible. Another sign was the performance of palliative amputation in patients with metastatic disease (14.5%) as a result of fungating lesions, pathologic fractures, or unmanageable pain. Results showed morbidity in 14.5%, and one patient died within 1 month of surgery, while others tolerated the surgery [58].

The typical medical practice for treating localized soft tissue sarcomas is limb-sparing surgery. Over the past three decades, the standard of care has changed from amputation to limb-sparing surgery and radiation therapy, with amputation occurring in less than 10% of cases [59].

The application of radiotherapy in the treatment of both localized and metastatic soft tissue sarcomas (STS) is widely recognized and accepted. Surgery combined with radiotherapy is the most efficient treatment for the majority of localized high-grade STS of the extremity, according to three randomized controlled trials. The 1982 National Cancer Institute experiment revealed that the survival rates for amputation and limb-sparing surgery were equal, establishing limb-sparing surgery in conjunction with radiotherapy as the new standard of practice. In the late 1990s, Yang et al. and Pisters et al. both looked at how adjuvant radiation affected local control in people with high-grade STS who had limb-sparing surgery compared to people who had no surgery [56].

Rosenberg et al., at the National Institutes of Health (NIH), conducted a study on the surgical treatment of STS in the extremities in 1982. A total of 43 patients were randomly randomized to either amputation (N = 16) or limb salvage with adjuvant external beam RT (N = 27) as treatment options. All patients received chemotherapy following surgery. The overall survival (OS) did not exhibit a significant disparity between the two groups, whereas the limb salvage group achieved a local control rate of 85%. The findings supported the practice of limb preservation, which has subsequently become a widely accepted standard of medical treatment [60].

4.1.2 Classification of surgical margins

Surgical margins are assessed and classified as radical, broad, marginal, and intralesional by the Musculo-Skeletal Tumor Society (MSTS) for both conservative resections and amputations (**Figure 6**) [10].

A marginal resection is the straightforward excision of the tumor and its pseudo capsule sometimes referred to as a "shell-out" or "whoops" procedure. After marginal resection, local recurrence rates can range from 50 to 93%. The fact that microscopic tumor cells can expand beyond the pseudo capsule and up to several centimeters beyond a palpable large tumor is not surprising. Marginal resection is not the proper course of action [62].

Intralesional resection: when dissecting into the lesion, the tumor's pseudo capsule has been breached and opened during surgery. Typically, microscopic, or macroscopic tumor tissue is left in the margins, and the exposed tissue planes may become contaminated. The most frequent intralesional procedures are subtotal "debulking" resections of the tumor or diagnostic incisional biopsies [62].

A broad resection: the terms "wide resection," "limb-sparing surgery," and "function-sparing surgery" are all used to refer to this procedure. En bloc excision of the tumor is required, along with the appropriate margin of normal tissue, which can range in width from a few centimeters to several, depending on the limitations of the anatomic structure. Although this treatment alone is typically associated with somewhat high local recurrence rates, ranging from 25 to 60%, it preserves reasonable function (limb salvage) [63].

The definition of adequate margin means margins of 2 cm or more with respect to anatomical barriers such as the periosteum or fascia [64]. It is generally agreed upon that surgical margins of less than 1.5 to 2 cm increase the chance of local recurrence. Unless further radiotherapy or surgery is done, if a surgical margin is inadequate and surrounded by an intact fascial layer or periosteum, this risk probably does not apply [43].

According to ESMO guidelines, the minimum margin on fixed tissue that should be regarded as adequate may vary depending on a number of variables, such as the histological subtype, preoperative treatments, and the presence of anatomical barriers such as fascia, vascular adventitia, periosteum, and epineurium [65].

Radical resection, which includes the amputation or removal of all the muscles and neurovascular structures within the compartment where the tumor is located. Local recurrence rates are substantially lower and vary from 0 to 18%. Although these local recurrence rates are acceptable, the cost of a limb (or a compartment) being lost is tremendous. Currently, amputations make up <5% of all sarcoma surgeries (**Figure 6**) [61, 66].

The American Joint Committee on Cancer (AJCC) classifies margins as negative (R0), microscopically positive (R1), or grossly positive (R2) using the R classification system [67].

The International Union Against Cancer (UICC) has recently modified the R classification to include the "R + 1 mm" classification, where the margin is designated as excessively positive (R2). In the past, specimens were classified as microscopically negative (R0) if there was a minimum of 1 mm of healthy tissue separating the tumor from the inked resection margin. Conversely, they were classified as microscopically positive (R1) if the tumor was located within 1 mm of the inked border. The UICC (R + 1 mm) classification's R0 margin standards are more stringent than those of the R classification [68].

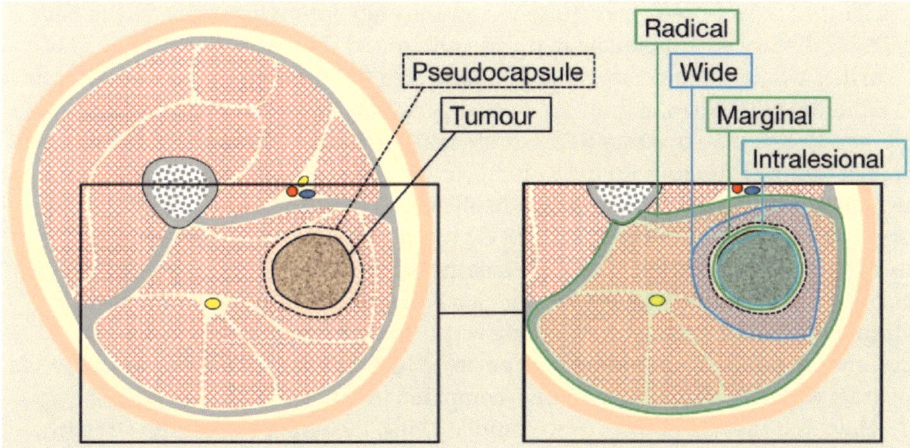

Figure 6.
Schematic diagram of soft tissue sarcoma excision. Cross-section of thigh showing tumor in adductor magnus with surrounding reactive zone, or "pseudo capsule." Four different classes of surgical excision are depicted, indicating the tissue excised with each type of resection [61].

The Toronto margin context classification (TMCC) identifies four categories of margins: negative margins (R0), unplanned positive margins, planned close margins with ultimately positive microscopic margins along critical structures, and positive margins resulting from tumor bed re-excision in patients initially treated with subpar surgery (the whoops procedure) [69].

4.2 Isolated limb perfusion

Locally advanced sarcomas or local recurrences are commonly treated with isolated limb perfusion. Few changes have been made to the treatment since it was adopted for treating sarcomas in 1992, following the addition of TNF. A significant component of the procedure is a 60-minute perfusion of melphalan and TNF under mild hyperthermia, which results in a 72 to 96% limb preservation rate, a 72 to 82.5% overall response rate, and acceptable toxicity according to the Wieberdink scale [70].

4.3 Adjuvant and neoadjuvant therapy for soft tissue sarcoma

4.3.1 Adjuvant radiotherapy

4.3.1.1 Limb sparing approach for localized extremity STS

Amputation was the standard of care for STS of the extremity until the results of the famous National Cancer Institute (NCI) randomized trial compared amputation to limb-sparing surgery plus postoperative radiation therapy in patients with high-grade STS of the extremity. They used a radiation dose of 50 Gy in a large volume, including the anatomic area at risk for local spread, followed by 10–20 Gy in a smaller volume of the tumor bed. Adjuvant chemotherapy was given to all patients. The trial showed comparable local control rates in both arms. Moreover, disease-free survival (DFS) and overall survival (OS) were not significantly different between the two arms. This trial proposed a new function-preserving option for patients who have a resectable disease with adequate margins and limited the use of amputation [71].

Further two randomized controlled trials tested the additional benefit of postoperative radiotherapy following limb-sparing surgery. The NCI randomized patients with high- and low-grade extremity STS to limb-sparing surgery alone or surgery followed by radiotherapy. Patients with high-grade sarcoma received adjuvant chemotherapy. The radiation was given in two phases. In phase I, a dose of 45 Gy was delivered to a large field, and then a boost dose of 18 Gy was given to the tumor bed. The trial found that adding radiation after limb-sparing surgery significantly decreased local recurrence, regardless of the grade. After a median follow-up of about 10 years, for high-grade STS, the local recurrence rate was 19% with surgery alone, with no local recurrence in the adjuvant radiotherapy arm. While for low-grade STS, the local recurrence rate was 33% after surgery alone, compared to 4% with adjuvant radiotherapy [72]. However, the rate of long-term complications, including worse limb strength, edema, and decreased range of motion, was higher in the radiotherapy arm.

A more recent updated report of the NCI study was published in 2014 with 20-year follow-up data concerning the quality of life. They found an increased rate of pathologic fracture, wound complications, and edema in the radiotherapy arm. In the same report, they confirmed a nonsignificantly better OS favoring adjuvant radiotherapy, although the trial was not powered to detect a survival difference [73].

In the other randomized trial, interstitial brachytherapy was in comparison to limb-sparing surgery alone. Brachytherapy was delivered using iridium-192 needles at a dose of 42–45 Gy over 4–6 days. After a median follow-up of about 6.3 years, they found a higher local recurrence rate in the surgery-only arm. For high-grade STS, the rate of local control was 66% with surgery alone, compared to 89% in the brachytherapy arm ($P = 0.0025$). In low-grade STS, adjuvant radiotherapy did not improve local control compared to surgery alone ($P = 0.49$). The trial also showed that adjuvant radiotherapy did not improve survival compared to surgery alone [74].

After a median follow-up of 100 months, a later update of this trial reported a 24% wound complication rate with adjuvant brachytherapy. Wound complications included reoperation for wound problems, wound separation greater than 2 cm, wound infection with purulent discharge, persistent seroma necessitating repeated aspirations, or hematoma formation volume of more than 25 mL. They reported an increased complication rate with large resection specimens [75].

Furthermore, a SEER database analysis found that patients with high-grade STS who received postoperative radiotherapy had better OS compared to surgery alone (HR 0.67, 95% CI 0.57–0.79). On the other hand, no OS benefit was found in patients with low-grade STS [76].

Although adjuvant radiotherapy improves local control over surgery alone, its value in small, low-grade tumors is questionable, especially when adequate tissue margins have been achieved following surgery [77]. A nomogram was made at MSKCC based on a study of recurrence rates among patients who had surgery without radiotherapy. This was done to make the decision of adjuvant radiotherapy more personalized. Five predictive factors were identified, including the patient's age, tumor size, grade, margin status, and histology [78].

4.3.1.2 Preoperative vs. postoperative radiotherapy

The use of preoperative radiotherapy before limb-sparing surgery was thought to be better than postoperative radiotherapy. For preoperative radiotherapy, a lower radiation dose to a smaller target volume is usually used, which may result in lower rates of long-term side effects. Preoperative radiotherapy may facilitate tumor resection by downsizing the tumor and decreasing the risk of microscopic tumor seeding during surgery. Moreover, delineating a well-visualized tumor volume is much easier than delineating a large area of the postoperative bed [79].

In a large Canadian trial, 190 patients were given either preoperative radiotherapy at a dose of 50 Gy in 25 fractions to the tumor plus a 2 cm expansion with a boost dose of 16 to 20 Gy after resection if the surgical margins were positive or postoperative radiotherapy at a dose of 66 Gy in 33 fractions. The wound complication rates were 35 and 17% in the preoperative and postoperative arms, respectively ($P = 0.01$). A higher rate of wound complications was seen in patients with lower extremities compared to patients with upper-extremity STS. Moreover, limb function at 6 weeks after surgery was worse in the preoperative arm ($P = 0.01$). At a median follow-up of 5 years, local control rates (93 vs. 92%) and OS (73 vs. 67%, $P = 0.48$) were equivalent in both arms [80].

A long-term evaluation of 129 patients found that limb function at 21 to 27 months after surgery was similar in both arms, but there was a statistical trend for more fibrosis, edema, and joint stiffness in the postoperative arm ($P = 0.07$) [81].

In general, preoperative radiotherapy is preferable, especially for large and/or high-grade STS, to downsize the tumor, decrease treated volumes, and facilitate surgical resection. Preoperative radiotherapy is also recommended for large radiosensitive STS subtypes like myxoid liposarcomas, which respond well to radiation compared to other histological subtypes [82].

4.3.1.3 Impact of margin status

Positive margin is a strong independent predictive factor of local recurrence, regardless of the use of adjuvant radiotherapy. Re-excision is usually indicated to clear margins after initially inadequate surgery. In a retrospective review, the data of 100 patients with high-grade sarcoma who had surgery with positive margins was analyzed. Local recurrence rates following surgery alone or surgery plus radiotherapy were 56 and 74%, respectively [83]. These local recurrence rates are higher than those observed in large series, in which most patients had clear resection margins. Even with the addition of adjuvant radiation, recurrence risk is still higher in the setting of positive margins. If a positive margin cannot be re-excised, a high radiation dose should be used up to 64 Gy due to statistically significant improvements in local control, disease-free survival, and overall survival [84].

4.3.1.4 Radiation therapy alone for unresectable disease

In patients who have initially unresectable disease, radiotherapy may be added for palliation of symptoms and to improve local control. An old study reported a 5-year local control rate of 33% in patients treated with external beam radiation therapy with doses ranging from 64 to 66 Gy [85]. An updated analysis from this study included 112 patients treated with definitive radiotherapy. They reported that the 5-year local control rate was dependent on tumor size and total dose. Regarding the tumor size, at 5 years, the local control rates were 51, 45, and 9% for tumors <5, 5–10, and > 10 cm, respectively. Regarding the total dose, the 5-year local control rate was 60% in patients who received >63 Gy, compared to 22% in patients receiving <63 Gy. The 5-year DFS and OS were also improved with higher doses. However, a higher complication rate was reported for higher doses >68 Gy (26 vs. 8%, $p = 0.02$) [86].

4.3.1.5 Radiotherapy techniques

External beam radiotherapy using 3D conformal radiotherapy (3DCRT) or intensity-modulated radiation therapy (IMRT) has been used as the gold standard radiotherapy technique. Other modalities, such as brachytherapy and intraoperative radiation therapy (IORT), decreased local recurrence after limb-sparing surgery. However, the local control rates are slightly lower than those reported with EBRT. The 5-year local control rates ranged from 82 to 84% with adjuvant brachytherapy [87]. A study comparing IMRT to brachytherapy found that IMRT improved 5-year local control rates in high-grade STS by 92% compared with 81% ($p = 0.04$) with brachytherapy. However, the major wound complications rate was 19% with IMRT compared to 11% with brachytherapy. While complications requiring reoperation were observed in 2% of patients treated with IMRT compared with 6% for those treated with brachytherapy [88].

This lower local control rate may be attributed to the smaller treated volume using brachytherapy and IORT alone, which may miss areas of subclinical disease or areas of extra compartmental spread. So, a hybrid treatment using brachytherapy, or IORT, as a boost in combination with EBRT was examined. Collectively, three series showed 5-year local control rates of 63–91.5% with wound healing complication rates of 12–34% [89–91].

4.3.2 Adjuvant and neoadjuvant chemotherapy

Although limb-sparing surgery preceded or followed by radiotherapy provided excellent long-term local control, up to 50% of patients with high-grade tumors will develop distant metastasis. So, the addition of adjuvant systemic chemotherapy to treat early micrometastatic disease gained a special interest in randomized trials and meta-analyses.

4.3.2.1 Randomized controlled trials of adjuvant chemotherapy

A single-agent doxorubicin was tested in the adjuvant setting in a large study conducted by the Scandinavian Sarcoma Group. After surgery +/− adjuvant radiotherapy, 240 patients were randomized to receive doxorubicin 60 mg/m^2 every 4 weeks for nine cycles or no chemotherapy. Data from 181 patients was available at the time of the analysis. After a median follow-up of about 40 months, single-agent doxorubicin did not improve local control, disease-free survival, or overall survival compared to the control arm. Further assessment of the survival data of the entire 240-patient cohort showed no difference in disease-free or overall survival between both treatment arms [92].

Combination chemotherapy for truncal and extremity soft tissue sarcomas was tested in a study by the Italian Sarcoma Study Group. After surgery +/− radiotherapy, 104 patients received either no chemotherapy or received ifosfamide (9 g/m^2 split over 5 days) and epirubicin (120 mg/m^2 split over 2 days) with filgrastim. Early termination of the study was decided after interim analysis, which showed that the primary endpoint of improved DFS was met. After a median follow-up of 36 months, OS was 72 vs. 55% in the chemotherapy arm and the no chemotherapy arm, respectively ($p = 0.002$). However, with longer follow-up, DFS did not reach a statistical significance level of $p = 0.05$, but 5-year overall survival was significantly better with chemotherapy [93]. This was the first study that showed a survival benefit for chemotherapy with ifosfamide-anthracycline-based therapy.

The EORTC conducted the largest randomized trial of adjuvant combination chemotherapy. The EORTC 62029 trial recruited 351 patients over 8 years. Patient characteristics were balanced between the treatment arms; about 47% of patients were > 50 years old, and about 54% were male. Histological subtypes included leiomyosarcoma 15%, liposarcoma 13%, MFH 11%, synovial 11%, with 60% of high-grade tumors, and two-thirds with an extremity primary. About 88% of patients received adjuvant radiotherapy. There was no significant survival benefit from adjuvant chemotherapy, with an equivalent 5-year DFS of 52% in both arms. The 5-year OS was comparable with 69% (observation) and 64% (chemotherapy) [94].

4.3.2.2 Meta-analyses of adjuvant chemotherapy

According to the Sarcoma Meta-analysis Collaboration (SMAC) group, data from different studies of adjuvant chemotherapy were put together in an old meta-analysis to make the case for using it stronger. They revised 23 studies but included 14 studies in the final analysis. Histological subtypes for each patient were reported but without a central pathological review. After a median follow-up of 9.4 years, 10-year DFS was superior to chemotherapy compared to no chemotherapy (55 vs. 45%, $p = 0.0001$). The 10-year local recurrence-free survival was also improved with chemotherapy (81 vs. 75%, $p = 0.016$). The 10-year OS was better with chemotherapy (54 vs. 50%), but not statistically significant ($p = 0.12$). A subgroup analysis of about 886 patients with extremity STS found a statistically significant improvement in overall survival: 46% of patients received chemotherapy compared to 39% of those who did not ($p = 0.029$) [95].

A more recent SMAC meta-analysis was published in 2008, which included modern studies using ifosfamide as part of adjuvant or neoadjuvant chemotherapy [96]. Most patients (about 95%) had STS in the extremity or trunk, where adequate surgical margins are most likely achieved. They reported a statistically significant reduction in local, distant, and overall recurrence for patients who received chemotherapy, compared to patients who did not receive chemotherapy. There was an absolute risk reduction of death of 6% (95% CI 2–11%; $p = 0.003$) favoring adjuvant chemotherapy. The 5-year survival rate was 46% for patients who received chemotherapy and 40% for those who did not. There were similar outcomes for patients who were treated in the ifosfamide-anthracycline-containing studies when analyzed alone or in combination with the older doxorubicin-based studies where ifosfamide was not used.

In conclusion, most individual clinical trials of adjuvant chemotherapy were negative. The encouraging results from the meta-analyses, however, might balance this. So, there is a small benefit from chemotherapy.

4.3.2.3 The patient selection for adjuvant chemotherapy

Based on the small benefit of adjuvant chemotherapy, defining a group of patients who may gain the biggest advantage from chemotherapy is critical. The chemosensitivity of different histological subtypes was not addressed in either meta-analyses or clinical trials, as no histological subtype represents the majority in any of these studies. Given the higher sensitivity of myxoid-round cell liposarcoma and synovial sarcoma to chemotherapy in metastatic soft tissue sarcoma (STS) compared to other subtypes, it is reasonable to anticipate potential benefits from adjuvant chemotherapy in individuals with these specific histological subtypes. A combined data analysis from two EORTC randomized trials of adjuvant therapy included 819 patients; no specific histological subtype gained a higher benefit from chemotherapy compared to others. In the same analysis, men appeared to benefit more than women, and patients under age 40 had worse outcomes than older patients, which is surprising since most patients under age 40 are diagnosed with chemotherapy-sensitive STS like synovial sarcoma and myxoid liposarcoma [97].

Two nomograms for predicting OS and distant metastases were developed based on retrospective data from 1452 extremity STS patients who had an operation at the Istituto Nazionale Tumori (Milan, Italy) from 1994 to 2013. The external validation of these nomograms was performed in three groups of patients from France, Canada, and the UK. The author confirmed the utility of these nomograms in predicting the risk of distant metastases and death after surgery. This information may help make decisions regarding the use of adjuvant chemotherapy in high-risk patients [98].

4.3.2.4 Neoadjuvant systemic chemotherapy

The role of neoadjuvant chemotherapy is debated, particularly for patients with large, unresectable, high-grade STS, to downsize the tumor. However, the data supporting the use of neoadjuvant chemotherapy for STS is scarce and mainly derived from retrospective series and small phase II trials [99, 100].

A new phase III RCT was done in Italy, France, and Poland to find out which is better for treating high-risk trunk and extremity STS: traditional anthracycline-ifosfamide-based neoadjuvant therapy or histology-based therapy. The study enrolled 287 patients who had nonmetastatic high-risk soft tissue sarcoma (STS) with a grade of 3 and a size of 5 cm or larger. These patients were classified into five histological subtypes: undifferentiated pleomorphic sarcoma (UPS) accounted for 33.8% of the cases, synovial sarcoma (SS) accounted for 24.4%, high-grade myxoid liposarcoma (HG-MLPS) accounted for 22.6%, leiomyosarcoma (LMS) accounted for 9.8%, and malignant peripheral nerve sheath tumor (MPNST) accounted for 9.4%. The control arm received three cycles of epirubicin 60 $mg/m^2/d$ short infusion for 2 days and ifosfamide 3 $g/m^2/d$ for 3 days. The investigational arm received histology-based regimens including gemcitabine 900 mg/m^2 on days 1 and 8 administered IV over 90 minutes, docetaxel 75 mg/m^2 on day 8 administered IV over 1 hour for UPS, The administration of ifosfamide at a high dosage of 14 g/m^2 is done over a period of 14 days using an external infusion pump for SS, trabectedin 1.3 mg/m^2, given by 24-hour continuous infusion for HG-MLPS, gemcitabine 1800 mg/m^2 on day 1 administered intravenously (IV) over 180 minutes, and dacarbazine 500 mg/m^2 on day 1 administered IV over 20 minutes for LMS, and etoposide 150 $mg/m^2/d$ on for 3 days and ifosfamide 3 $g/m^2/d$ on days for 3 days for MPNST. After a median follow-up of 52 months, there was no difference in 5-year DFS and OS, and no treatment-related deaths were observed between both arms [101].

The Japanese JCOG1306 phase II/III randomized trial compared gemcitabine-docetaxel to standard adriamycin-ifosfamide and concluded that the anthracycline-ifosfamide combination should still be the standard regimen for neoadjuvant chemotherapy in high-risk extremity and trunk STSS [102].

In the absence of strong evidence, a multidisciplinary team discussion is essential to select patients for neoadjuvant chemotherapy. Patient factors, such as age and comorbidity, together with the tumor characteristics, including histology, subtype, stage, and resectability, should all be considered in discussing the appropriateness of this approach on a case-by-case basis.

4.3.3 Special consideration for retroperitoneal STS

Retroperitoneal sarcomas (RPS) pose several challenges in management. They are a group of rare, heterogeneous tumors that often present with large masses. The risk of complete surgical eradication is high due to its critical proximity to abdominal organs. So, the local recurrence rate is higher than the extremity and trunk STS. Local recurrence rates are common with high-grade tumors and following macroscopically incomplete resections [103].

4.3.3.1 Adjuvant radiotherapy

Pre- or postoperative EBRT and/or IORT are usually used in combination with surgery to decrease the risk of local recurrence. Several retrospective database studies confirmed the positive impact of preoperative or postoperative radiotherapy on survival compared to surgery alone. A US National Cancer Data Base study investigated the added role of preoperative compared to surgery alone in retroperitoneal liposarcoma. Preoperative radiotherapy followed by resection improved survival compared to surgery alone, with a median overall survival of 129.2 versus 84.3 months, respectively ($P = 0.046$). The effect of preoperative radiotherapy on survival was more apparent in large, advanced tumors with organ invasion. The median overall survival was not reached in the preoperative radiotherapy cohort versus 63.8 months in the surgery-only cohort ($P = 0.044$) [104].

A separate case-control study examined a cohort of 9068 individuals diagnosed with localized retroperitoneal sarcoma, sourced from a comprehensive clinical oncology database, and who had treatment between 2003 and 2011. Both preoperative and postoperative radiotherapy were significantly linked to a better overall survival rate (OS) compared to surgery alone [105].

Preoperative radiotherapy is usually preferred over postoperative radiotherapy since radiation enteritis is significantly lower as the tumor mass displaces the small intestine away from the radiation beam. Moreover, it is easier to treat a small tumor volume than a large operative bed. A radiation dose of 45 to 50 Gy is recommended for preoperative radiotherapy. VMAT or IMRT, is vastly superior to 3DCRT in terms of radiation dose homogeneity and dose to organs at risk [106].

The latest phase III randomized STRASS trial (EORTC-62092) revealed that preoperative radiation does not provide therapeutic benefits for retroperitoneal sarcoma. The study comprised a cohort of 266 patients diagnosed with nonmetastatic retroperitoneal soft tissue sarcoma (STS). Its objective was to examine the effect of combining preoperative radiation with surgery, as opposed to surgery alone, on the rate of abdominal recurrence-free survival. The administration of radiotherapy involved delivering a total dose of 50·4 Gy in 28 fractions, utilizing either 3DCRT or IMRT techniques. This was followed by the surgical removal of the tumor mass, ensuring complete removal of the visible tumor along with the adjacent organs if required. Following a median follow-up period of 43.1 months, the projected median duration of survival without abdominal recurrence was 4.5 years in the group that had radiotherapy in addition to surgery and 5.0 years in the group that underwent surgery alone. The hazard ratio was 1.01, with a 95% confidence interval of 0.71–1.44. The log rank p-value was 0.95. Higher toxicity was also seen in the radiotherapy arm [107].

4.3.3.2 Adjuvant chemotherapy

Most of the trials addressing the role of postoperative chemotherapy have been performed in the setting of advanced-extremity STS. Data to support the usability of chemotherapy following resection in retroperitoneal STS is very limited, and the extrapolation of data from extremity trials may not be appropriate. Since mortality in RPS often occurs in the absence of distant metastases, the priority should be eliminating the risk of local recurrence. The use of preoperative chemotherapy alone or in combination with radiotherapy was tested in several studies.

An Italian study reported on the long-term outcomes of 83 patients treated with neoadjuvant high-dose long-infusion ifosfamide along with preoperative radiotherapy followed by surgery for localized retroperitoneal STS. About 72% of the patients completed the neoadjuvant chemoradiotherapy regimen. With 91.7 months of median follow-up, the DFS and OS were 46.6 and 63.2% at 7 years, respectively. This study confirmed the long-term feasibility and safety of this approach [108].

A NCD analysis study included patients with localized retroperitoneal STS who received different regimens of pre- or postoperative chemotherapy. The study showed a worse median OS in the chemotherapy group compared to surgery alone (40 vs. 68.2 months; $p < 0.01$). Even after propensity score matching, lower OS in the chemotherapy group persisted (40 vs. 52.4 months; $p = 0.002$). However, it is difficult to draw firm conclusions from these data since patients with large, high-grade tumors were more likely to receive chemotherapy [109].

In conclusion, the available data in retroperitoneal STS demonstrated the feasibility of preoperative chemotherapy or chemoradiotherapy. However, there are concerns about toxicity, which may interfere with the patient's definitive surgical treatment afterward. So, preoperative treatment may be considered in borderline resectable tumors, particularly in high-grade, relatively chemo-sensitive subtypes such as leiomyosarcomas, undifferentiated pleomorphic sarcomas, and grade 3 dedifferentiated liposarcomas [110].

5. Systemic therapies in advanced and metastatic soft tissue sarcoma

Since the first studies in the 1970s, doxorubicin has been and remains the single most active agent for the treatment of STS. There is much variation in its reported response rate given the underlying tumor heterogeneity of early trials, which predominantly included multiple STS subtypes. Modern-day studies in unselected STS reported response rates of 10–25% [111].

It is important to recognize that there is a dose-response relationship with doxorubicin, seen at doses between 60 and 75 mg/m^2 per cycle [112]. Other agents have been investigated to try and avoid dose-limiting cumulative cardiotoxicity [113]. Epirubicin has an equal dose, less cardiotoxicity, and a similar toxicity profile and response rate. However, most of the data were collected using doxorubicin, so in most parts of the world, doxorubicin is still the more well-known treatment. Alternatively, liposomal doxorubicin, in phase II studies, has similar activity to doxorubicin with response rates between 10 and 50% and an improved toxicity profile [114].

Multiple randomized trials have looked at the combination of doxorubicin and ifosfamide, but they have not found any clear, useful evidence to show that the combination approach is better than using doxorubicin alone. While these combinations are associated with higher response rates (range of 15–46%) when compared with single-agent doxorubicin (10–18%), they have not improved overall survival. Moreover, toxicity was significantly greater for the combination group [115, 116].

So, the choice of combination versus single-agent therapy in the first line must be designed exclusively for the patient, suggesting that the combination may have a role to play in selected patients where tumor shrinkage is an important goal of treatment, for example, neoadjuvant chemotherapy, or in patients with highly symptomatic lesions but minimal other comorbidities, allowing them to tolerate a more aggressive approach [43].

The GeDDiS trial was a phase 3 randomized controlled trial performed at 24 institutions in the UK and one hospital connected with the Swiss Group for Clinical Cancer Research (SAKK). Patients needed to have histologically proven locally advanced or metastatic soft tissue sarcoma and have never received doxorubicin or sarcoma treatment before. Patients were given either six cycles of doxorubicin or six cycles of gemcitabine/docetaxel at random. Results showed that gemcitabine/docetaxel was not superior to doxorubicin for either PFS or OS, so it can be an alternative when anthracycline is clinically contraindicated [117].

More recently, LMS-04, a randomized multicenter phase III trial that included 150 patients from 20 centers of the French Sarcoma Group, compared doxorubicin alone to doxorubicin and trabectedin as first-line therapy for advanced leiomyosarcoma. Inclusion criteria were patients with age >/= 18 years old, ECOG 0-1, metastatic or unresectable leiomyosarcoma of soft tissue or uterine, who had not received chemotherapy before. Doxorubicin/trabectedin in first-line therapy increased PFS compared to doxorubicin alone and could be considered as a first-line treatment for metastatic leiomyosarcoma [118].

5.1 Second-line systemic therapies

Other systemic medications are thought of as second-line medications. Gemcitabine is effective in treating refractory STS and more effective in treating leiomyosarcoma, angiosarcoma, and, to some extent, pleomorphic sarcoma. There is conflicting evidence on the benefits of a gemcitabine dacarbazine GD regimen over gemcitabine alone, despite its higher tolerability in a palliative setting [119].

In terms of PFS, OS, and RR, gemcitabine with docetaxel is more successful than gemcitabine alone, but with higher toxicity. Phase II studies of the combination showed an overall response rate as high as 53%. In uterine leiomyosarcomas, studies including other soft tissue sarcomas showed a response rate of 14–53% [120].

Trabectedin is an alkylating agent (a tetrahydroisoquinoline alkaloid) that is thought to work by attaching to the minor groove of DNA and damaging the machinery that fixes DNA nucleotides. It is suggested for people who did not respond to anthracycline-based therapy [121]. A PFS of 3.3 months and an overall survival of 13.9 months were found in research on trabectedin 24-hour infusion. These studies' findings led to the approval of trabectedin for treatment in patients who had progressed on doxorubicin or ifosfamide in Europe in 2007, particularly in cases with myxoid liposarcoma and leiomyosarcoma, so-called "histocyte-specific cytotoxic agents" [122].

Another example of histocyte-specific cytotoxicity in patients with advanced STS is eribulin, a microtubule inhibitor. In a phase II study, the EORTC examined the efficacy of eribulin in people with adipocytic, leiomyosarcoma, and synovial sarcomas. Eribulin 1.4 mg/m^2 was administered to 115 patients on days 1 and 8 of a 21-day cycle for analysis and treatment. Patients with leiomyosarcoma had a PFS of 31.6%, those with adipocytic sarcoma had a PFS of 46.9%, and those with synovial sarcoma had a PFS of 21.1% at 12 weeks. Patients with adipocytic sarcomas had a median PFS of 2.6 months, whereas those with leiomyosarcoma and synovial sarcoma had median PFS of 2.9 months each [123]. Patients with advanced liposarcoma and leiomyosarcoma who received eribulin had longer overall survival (OS) than those who received dacarbazine in a phase 3 trial (13.5 vs. 11.5 months, respectively; P = 0.0169). Patients with liposarcoma had the greatest benefit (median OS, 15.6 vs. 8.4). Median PFS was comparable in both treatment groups (2.6 months) [124].

5.2 Tyrosine kinase inhibitors (TKIs) or multi-targeted kinase inhibitors

TKIs are small, multifunctional molecules that induce downstream effects such as inhibition of angiogenesis, cell growth, and proliferation.

Pazopanib was the first targeted substance to be approved in non-GIST STS and was indicated in patients who had demonstrated poor response to earlier chemotherapy. In an early EORTC study, 62,043 was conducted for Pazopanib in patients with relapsed or refractory advanced soft tissue sarcoma. In total, 140 patients with intermediate- or high-grade soft tissue sarcoma were enrolled, including adipocytic STS, leiomyosarcoma, synovial sarcoma, and other STS types. Results showed that pazopanib was well tolerated in patients with relapsed, advanced STS but had insufficient activity on the liposarcoma subtype [125].

The Spanish Sarcoma Group and the German interdisciplinary Sarcoma Group established a phase II trial (NCT01692496) to monitor the activity of pazopanib on liposarcoma in two cohort groups: well-differentiated or dedifferentiated liposarcoma and myxoid or round-cell liposarcoma. Results showed that pazopanib was well tolerated in well-differentiated and dedifferentiated subtypes but not in myxoid liposarcoma [126].

A phase II trial was established by the Spanish Sarcoma Group and the German interdisciplinary Sarcoma Group (NCT01692496) that was designed to observe the activity of pazopanib on liposarcoma in two cohort groups: well-differentiated differentiated/dedifferentiated liposarcoma and myxoid or round-cell liposarcoma. Results showed that pazopanib was well tolerated in well-differentiated and dedifferentiated subtypes, but not in myxoid liposarcoma [127].

The EPAZ trial showed that pazopanib was just as effective as doxorubicin in treating STS in older patients. This suggests that pazopanib could be used as the first treatment for STS in people aged 60 and up. There was superiority with pazopanib in terms of neutropenia and febrile neutropenia in elderly patients with STS. The overall incidence of toxicity remained similar for both treatments, but there were differences in the AE profiles that may help tailor treatment to individual needs in this population [128].

5.3 Immune checkpoint inhibitors (ICIs)

A treatment option for individuals with advanced and metastatic cancer is pembrolizumab, an anti-PD-1 antibody that exhibits encouraging action in undifferentiated sarcomas [129].

Studies have also been done on the effects of pembrolizumab and nivolumab, two humanized monoclonal IgG4 antibodies that target the PD-1 cell surface receptor. These antibodies may be used alone or in combination with cytotoxic and antiangiogenic medications. In the SARC028 phase 2 study, pembrolizumab worked well as a single drug for all types of undifferentiated STS, with an ORR of 17.5 and a 55% 3-month PFS. Undifferentiated pleomorphic sarcoma and dedifferentiated liposarcoma seemed to benefit the most [130].

Patients with alveolar soft part sarcoma (ASPS) showed outstanding outcomes with ICIs. A single-center phase II study with axitinib and pembrolizumab was presented by Wilky and colleagues. Eleven of the patients had been diagnosed with ASPS. Six (54.5%) of the 11 patients showed an objective response, and the median PFS was 12.4 months (95% CI, 2.7–22.3) [131].

5.4 Systemic treatment for certain benign or malignant soft tissue tumors

Because we know more about the different types of STS histology and because of the results of many retrospective reviews and prospective randomized studies, it is important to treat these types of histology with care [132].

- *Angiosarcoma* is highly sensitive to taxanes. Gemcitabine is an alternative, either as a single agent or in combination with docetaxel [133].

- *Perivascular epithelioid cell tumor (PEComa)* is a family of rare mesenchymal tumors consisting of perivascular epithelioid cells. TSC1 and TSC2 mutations disrupting the mTOR signaling pathway led to the exploration of mTOR inhibitors in PEComas [134]. Activity of sirolimus and temsirolimus has been reported in small case series [135].

- *Dermatofibrosarcoma protuberans (DFSP):* Imatinib is the usual first-line medicinal treatment [136]. DFSPs are characterized by a unique translocation t (17;22) (q22; q13), resulting in the COL1A1/PDGFB fusion gene, responsible for platelet-derived growth factor beta receptor activation, hence the imatinib activity [137].

- *Desmoid tumors DTFs* are benign fibroblastic proliferations characterized by infiltrative growth. There are two different types of DTF that have been described: sporadic DTF linked to the CTNNB1 mutation and DTF linked to the APC germline mutation. Wnt/APC/β-catenin pathway alterations are considered to be the drivers of tumor proliferation [138]. For those who fail the "wait and see" management, pazopanib, and sorafenib showed activity with a good response rate in progressive symptomatic patients [139, 140]. Also, there are better data for liposomal doxorubicin, single-agent vinorelbine, and combination methotrexate/vinorelbine or methotrexate/vinblastine [141, 142]. More recently, nirogacestat is an oral, specific, and small-molecule gamma-secretase inhibitor. There was a statistically significant improvement in the risk of disease progression in patients who were randomly assigned to nirogacestat compared to placebo in a DeFi study. On average, the risk of disease progression dropped by 71% [143].

- *Pigmented villonodular synovitis (PVNS)*, otherwise known as tenosynovial giant cell tumor, is a rare but well-recognized proliferative disorder of synovial tissue.

It is considered a benign neoplasm, lacking malignant and metastatic potential. A translocation in *CSF1-COL6A3*, t (1;2) (p13; q35), leads to overexpression of the colony-stimulating factor 1 receptor (CSF1R) [144]. Imatinib and nilotinib showed some CSF1R inhibitor activity [145]. The more potent CSF1R inhibitor, pexidartinib, showed an impressive overall response rate but also had significant hepatic toxicity [144].

- *Solitary fibrous tumor (SFT):* the more potent CSF1R inhibitor, pexidartinib, showed an impressive overall response rate but also had significant hepatic toxicity [146]. Anti-angiogenetic agents such as pazopanib, sunitinib, and sorafenib are shown to be active in this entity [147]. It tends to be refractory to doxorubicin, but there has been a variable response seen with other cytotoxic agents, including dacarbazine and trabectedin [148].

- Alveolar soft part sarcoma (ASPS) is a rare subtype of soft tissue sarcoma (STS) that is caused by a specific genetic abnormality known as t(X;17) (p11; q25) translocation. ASPS is known for its slow-growing nature, yet it tends to spread to the lungs and brain. It is regarded as inherently resistant to chemotherapy. Tyrosine kinase inhibitors, including sunitinib, cediranib, and pazopanib, have demonstrated efficacy in over 50% of instances, resulting in tumor responses or disease stability [149]. Immune checkpoint inhibitors have also shown promising activity in ASPS based on early-phase immunotherapy trials [150].

- *Endometrial stromal sarcoma (ESS)* Low-grade ESS is the most common subtype of ESS. They are indolent tumors characterized by strong expression of the hormone receptors CD10 and Bcl2. At a molecular level, *JAZF1* rearrangements are common and are regarded as diagnostic [151]. They are highly sensitive to progestins, such as medroxyprogesterone (Provera), and hormonal therapy is preferred over cytotoxic agents in the first line. Chemotherapeutic agents are generally reserved for patients with hormone-resistant diseases [152]. High-grade ESS has an aggressive natural history, is characterized by a lack of hormone receptor and CD10 expression, and may have a translocation that results [153].

6. Conclusion

Soft tissue sarcoma (STS) is a group of diseases with varying biological characteristics and particular responses to treatment based on their location and histological type, rather than a single entity. Surgery is the primary treatment for limited primary disease. The strategy that is advised is to undergo scheduled surgery with the objective of achieving microscopically negative margins. Neoadjuvant and/or adjuvant chemotherapy and radiation therapy are frequently employed to enhance treatment outcomes and optimize the quality of surgical margins although emerging research is showing the importance of using multiple treatment methods for these tumors. To optimize patient care, it is imperative that cases be deliberated upon in a multidisciplinary team (MDT) setting. Furthermore, treatment strategies should be tailored to the individual patient, considering a comprehensive understanding of the distinct behavioral patterns exhibited by specific pathologic types, with particular emphasis on infiltrative variants.

Acronyms and abbreviations

AJCC	American Joint Committee on Cancer
ASCO	American Society of Clinical Oncolog
STSs	soft tissue sarcomas
LFS	Li-Fraumeni syndrome
FAP	familial adenomatous polyposis
RAS	radiation-associated sarcoma
US	ultrasound
CT	computed tomography
CNB	core needle biopsy
IHC	immunohistochemistry
TKIs	tyrosine kinase inhibitors
JCO.	Journal of Clinical Oncology
ICIs	immune checkpoint inhibitors
PEComa	perivascular epithelioid cell tumor
DFSP	dermatofibrosarcoma protuberans
DFT	desmoid tumor
APC	the adenomatous polyposis coli

Author details

Mohamed Kelany[1*], Ahmed R. Eldesoky[2], Asmaa A. Abdeltawab[3]
and Noha Mohamed[1]

1 Clinical Oncology, Ain Shams University, Cairo, Egypt

2 Clinical Oncology, Mansoura University, Cairo, Egypt

3 Clinical Oncology, Assuit University, Cairo, Egypt

*Address all correspondence to: kelaney.m@med.asu.edu.eg

References

[1] Zhang P, Brooks JS. Modern pathological evaluation of soft tissue sarcoma specimens and its potential role in soft tissue sarcoma research. Current Treatment Options in Oncology [Internet]. 2004;**5**(6):441-450. Available from: http://www.ncbi.nlm.nih.gov/pubmed/1550

[2] Halperin EC, Wazer DE, Perez CA, Brady LW. Perez and Brady's: Principles and Practice of Radiation Oncology. 5th ed. 2008. pp. 1803-1821

[3] Siegel RL, Miller KD, Jemal A. Cancer statistics. CA: A Cancer Journal for Clinicians. 2022;**72**(1):7-33

[4] Stiller CA, Tram A, Serriano D, Rossi S, et al. Descriptive epidemiology of sarcomas in Europe: Report from the RARECARE project. European Journal of Cancer [Internet]. 2013;**49**(3):684-695. Available from: http://www.ncbi.nlm.nih.gov/pubmed/

[5] Gage MM, Nagarajan N, Ruck JM, et al. Sarcomas in the United States: Recent trends and a call for improved staging. Oncotarget. 2019;**10**:2462-2474

[6] Dennis NM, Lawrence G. Soft tissue sarcoma incidence and survival tumours diagnosed in England between 1985 and 2009. Report number R12/06; London. 2012

[7] Toro JR, Travis LB, WU HJ, et al. Incidence patterns of soft tissue sarcomas, regardless of primary site, in the surveillance, epidemiology and end results program, 1978 – 2001: An analysis of 26, 758 cases. International Journal of Cancer. 2006;**119**(2922-2930):2927

[8] Smith AW, Bellizzi KM, Keegan TH, et al. Health-related quality of life of adolescent and young adult patients with cancer in the United States: The adolescent and young adult health outcomes and patient experience study. Journal of Clinical Oncology. 2013;**31**(17):2136-2145

[9] Sangkhathat S et al. Current management of pediatric soft tissue sarcomas. World Journal of Clinical Pediatrics. 2015;**4**(4):94-105

[10] Hung G-Y, Horng J-L, Chen PC-H, et al. Incidence of soft tissue sarcoma in Taiwan: A nationwide population-based study (2007-2013). Cancer Epidemiology. 2019;**60**:185-192

[11] Li FP, Fraumeni JF, Mulvihill JJ, et al. A cancer family syndrome in twenty-four kindreds. Cancer Research. 1988;**48**(18):5358-5362

[12] Correa H. Li-Fraumeni syndrome. Journal of Pediatric Genetics. 2016;**5**(2):84-88. DOI: 10.1055/s-0036-1579759. Epub 2016 Apr 13

[13] Ognjanovic S, Olivier M, Bergemann, et al. Sarcomas in TP53 germline mutation carriers: A review of the IARC TP53 database. Cancer. 2012;**118**(5):1387

[14] Groen EJ, Roos A, Muntinghe FL, et al. Extra-intestinal manifestations of familial adenomatous polyposis. Annals of Surgical Oncology. 2008;**15**(9):2439-2450

[15] Wong JR, Morton LM, Tucker MA, et al. Risk of subsequent malignant neoplasms in long-term hereditary retinoblastoma survivors after chemotherapy and radiotherapy. Journal of Clinical Oncology. 2008;**32**(29):3284-3290

[16] Colman SD, Wiliams CA, Wallac MR, et al. Benign neurofibromas in type

1 neurofibromatosis (NF1) show somatic deletions of the NF1 gene. Nature Genetics. 1995;**11**(1):90-92. DOI: 10.1038/ng0995-90

[17] Ducatman BS, Scheithauer BW, Piepgras DG, et al. Malignant peripheral nerve sheath tumors. A clinicopathologic study of 120 cases. Cancer. 1986;**57**(10):2006-2021. DOI: 10.1002/1097-0142(19860515)57:10<2006::aid-cncr2820571022>3.0.co;2-6

[18] Fletcher JA, Kozakewich HP, Hoffer FA, et al. Diagnostic relevance of clonal cytogenetic aberrations in malignant soft-tissue tumors. The New England Journal of Medicine. 1991;**324**(7):436-442

[19] MacConaill LE, Garcia E, Shivdasani P, et al. Prospective enterprise-level molecular genotyping of a cohort of cancer patients. The Journal of Molecular Diagnostics. 2014;**16**(6):660-672

[20] Mariño-Enríquez A, Bovee JV. Molecular pathogenesis and diagnostic, prognostic and predictive molecular markers in sarcoma. Surgical Pathology Clinics. 2016;**9**(3):457-473. DOI: 10.1016/j.path.2016.04.009

[21] Murray EM, Werner D, Greef EA, et al. Postradiation sarcomas: 20 cases and a literature review. International Journal of Radiation Oncology, Biology, Physics. 1999;**45**:951-961

[22] Negishi T, Matsunobu A, Endo M, et al. An analysis of 20 cases of radiation-associated sarcoma, including 4 cases treated by carbon ion radiotherapy. Oncology. 2022;**100**(3):148-154

[23] Mundt KA, Dell LD, Crawford L, et al. Quantitative estimated exposure to vinyl chloride and risk of angiosarcoma of the liver and hepatocellular cancer in the US industry-wide vinyl chloride cohort: Mortality update through 2013. Occupational and Environmental Medicine. 2017;**74**(10):oemed-2016-104051

[24] Xu J, Ye Y, Huang F, et al. Association between dioxin and cancer incidence and mortality: A meta-analysis. Scientific Reports. 2016;**6**:38012

[25] Schulte M, Von Bear A, Schultheiss M, et al. Sonografische Klassifikation solider WeichteiltumorenGerman. Classification of solid soft tissue tumours by ultrasonography. Ultraschall in der Medizin. 2010;**31**(2):182-190. DOI: 10.1055/s-0028-1109917

[26] Aga P, Singh R, Parihar A, et al. Imaging spectrum in soft tissue sarcomas. Indian Journal of Surgical Oncology. 2011;**2**(4):271-279. DOI: 10.1007/s13193-011-0095-1 Epub 2011 Dec 10

[27] Papp DF, JKhanna AJ, McCarthy EF, et al. Magnetic resonance imaging of soft-tissue tumors: Determinate and indeterminate lesions. The Journal of Bone and Joint Surgery. American Volume. 2007;**89**(3):103-115

[28] Dourmishev LA, Dourmishev AL, Lukac DM, et al. Molecular genetics of Kaposi's sarcoma-associated herpesvirus (human herpesvirus-8) epidemiology and pathogenesis. Microbiology and Molecular Biology Reviews : MMBR. 2003;**67**(2):175-212. table of contents. doi: 10.1

[29] Shon W, Ida CM, Boland-Froemming JM, et al. Cutaneous angiosarcoma arising in massive localized lymphedema of the morbidly obese: A report of five cases and review of the literature. Journal of Cutaneous Pathology. 2011

[30] Soper JR, Brown WE, Schatz JA, et al. Radiology of bone and soft

tissue sarcomas. Cancer Forum. 2010;**34**:126-130

[31] Spinnato P, Roberta C, et al. MRI tail sign in soft-tissue sarcoma. Reviews and Commentary Images in Radiology. 2021. DOI: 10.1148/radiol.2021203877

[32] Scalas G, Parmeggiani A. Magnetic resonance imaging of soft tissue sarcoma: Features related to prognosis. European Journal of Orthopaedic Surgery and Traumatology. 2021;**31**(8):1567-1575. DOI: 10.1007/s00590-021-0

[33] Carvalho K, Cunch I, Rocha R, et al. GLUT1 expression in malignant tumors and its use as an immunodiagnostic marker. Clinics (São Paulo, Brazil). 2011;**66**:965-997

[34] Rakheja R, Makis W, Tulbah R, et al. Necrosis on FDG PET/CT correlates with prognosis and mortality in sarcomas. AJR. American Journal of Roentgenology. 2013;**201**:170-177

[35] Macpherson RE, Pratap S, Tyrrell H, et al. Retrospective audit of 957 consecutive 18F-FDG PET-CT scans compared to CT and MRI in 493 patients with different histological subtypes of bone and soft tissue sarcoma. Clinical Sarcoma Research. 2018;**8**(1):9

[36] Suzuki R, Watanabe H, Yanagava T, et al. PET evaluation of fatty tumors in the extremity: Possibility of using the standardized uptake value (SUV) to differentiate benign tumors from liposarcoma. Annals of Nuclear Medicine. 2005;**19**(8):661-670

[37] Brenner W, Eary JF, Hwang w, et al. Risk assessment in liposarcoma patients based on FDG PET imaging. European Journal of Nuclear Medicine and Molecular Imaging. 2006;**33**:1290-1295

[38] Lucas JD, O'Dohetry MJ, Wong JC, et al. Evaluation of fluorodeoxyglucose positron emission tomography in the management of soft tissue sarcomas. Journal of Bone and Joint Surgery. British Volume (London). 1998;**80**(3):441-447

[39] Volker T, Denecke T, Steffen I, et al. Positron emission tomography for staging of pediatric sarcoma patients: Results of a prospective multicenter trial. Journal of Clinical Oncology. 2007;**25**:5435-5441

[40] Ricard SF, Cimarelli S, Deshayes E, Choong PF, et al. Additional benefit of F-18 FDG PET/CT in the staging and follow-up of pediatric rhabdomyosarcoma. Clinical Nuclear Medicine. 2011;**36**:672

[41] Strauss DC, Thway K, Fisher C, Thomas JM, et al. The role of core needle biopsy in the diagnosis of suspected soft tissue tumours. Journal of Surgical Oncology. 2010;**102**:523-529. DOI: 10.1002/jso.21600

[42] Strauss DC, Qureshi YA, Thomas JM, et al. The role of core needle biopsy in the diagnosis of suspected soft tissue tumours. Journal of Surgical Oncology. 2010;**102**:523-529. DOI: 10.1002/jso.21600

[43] Choong PFM. Sarcoma a Practical Guide to Multidisciplinary Management. Austria; 2021. ISBN 978-981-15-9413-7. ISBN 978-981-15-9414-4 (eBook). DOI: 10.1007/978-981-15-9414-4

[44] Wu JS, Goldsmith JD, Hochman MG, et al. Bone and soft-tissue lesions: What factors affect diagnostic yield of image-guided core-needle biopsy? Radiology. 2008;**248**:962-970. DOI: 10.1148/radiol.2483071742

[45] Garcia del Muro X, de Alava E, Artigas V, et al. Clinical practice guidelines for the diagnosis and treatment of patients with soft tissue sarcoma by the

Spanish group for research in sarcomas (GEIS). Cancer Chemotherapy and Pharmacology. 2016;**77**(1):133-146

[46] Kim SY, Chung HW, Tack Sun O, et al. Practical guidelines for ultrasound-guided core needle biopsy of soft-tissue lesions: Transformation from beginner to specialist. Korean Journal of Radiology. 2017;**18**(2):361-369

[47] Lindberg MR. Diagnostic Pathology: Soft Tissue Tumors. Amsterdam: Elsevier Health Sciences; 2015

[48] Kuhn KJ, Cloutier JM, Boutin, et al. Soft tissue pathology for the radiologist: A tumor board primer with 2020 WHO classification update. Skeletal Radiology;**2021**. DOI: 10.1007/s00256-020-03567-

[49] Weiss SW, Enzinger FM. Malignant fibrous histiocytoma: An analysis of 200 cases. Cancer. 1978;**41**(6):2250-2266

[50] Fletcher CD. Pleomorphic malignant fibrous histiocytoma: Fact or fiction? A critical reappraisal based on 159 tumors diagnosed as pleomorphic sarcoma. The American Journal of Surgical Pathology. 1992;**16**(3):213-228

[51] Wang L, Ren W, Wang J, et al. Pleomorphic liposarcoma: A clinicopathological, immunohistochemical and molecular cytogenetic study of 32 additional cases. Pathology International. 2013;**63**(11):523-531

[52] Maki RG, Moraco N, Antonescu CR, et al. Toward better soft tissue sarcoma staging: Building on American joint committee on cancer staging systems versions 6 and 7. Annals of Surgical Oncology. 2013;**20**:3377-3383

[53] Cates JMM. The AJCC 8th edition staging system for soft tissue sarcoma of the extremities or trunk: A cohort study of the SEER database. Journal of the National Comprehensive Cancer Network. 2018;**16**(2):144-152

[54] Italiano A, Di Mauro I, Rapp J, et al. Clinical effect of molecular methods in sarcoma diagnosis (GENSARC): A prospective, multicentre, observational study. The Lancet Oncology. 2016;**17**(4):532

[55] Guadagnolo BA, Xu Y, Zagars GK, et al. A population-based study of the quality of care in the diagnosis of large (≥5 cm) soft tissue sarcomas. American Journal of Clinical Oncology. 2012;**35**:455-461

[56] Vodanovich DA, Choong MPF. Soft-tissue sarcomas. Indian Journal of Orthopaedics. 2018;**52**(1):35-44

[57] Parsons CM, Pimiento JM, Cheong D, et al. The role of radical amputations for extremity tumors: A single institution experience and review of the literature. Journal of Surgical Oncology. 2012;**105**(2):149-155

[58] Smith HG, Thomas JM, Smith MJF, et al. Major amputations for extremity soft-tissue sarcoma. Annals of Surgical Oncology. 2017. DOI: 10.1245/s10434-017-5895-2

[59] Windhager R, Hobusch GM. The role of surgery in soft tissue sarcoma: Can we improve outcome and function towards sporting activities?. Memo-Magazine of European. Medical Oncology. 2020;**13**(2):164-168

[60] MacNeill AJ, Gupta A, Swallow CJ. Randomized controlled trials in soft tissue sarcoma: We are getting there! Surgical Oncology Clinics of North America. 2017;**26**(4):531-544

[61] Steele A, Ashford, et al. Surgical management of soft tissue sarcoma.

Orthopaedics and Traumatology. 2017;**31**(3):180-187. DOI: 10.1016/j.mporth.2017.03.012

[62] Capanna R, Frenos F. Surgery for soft tissue sarcomas. In: Bentley G, editor. European Surgical Orthopaedics and Traumatology. Berlin, Heidelberg: Springer; 2014. DOI: 10.1007/978-3-642-34746-7_218

[63] Bagaria SP, Chang YH, Gray RJ, et al. Improving long-term outcomes for patients with extra-abdominal soft tissue sarcoma regionalization to high-volume centers, improved compliance with guidelines or both? Sarcoma. 2018:8141056. DOI: 10.1155/2018/8141056

[64] Kawaguchi N, Ahmed AR, Matsushita Y, et al. The concept of curative margin in surgery for bone and soft tissue sarcoma. Clinical Orthopaedics and Related Research. 2004;**419**:165-172

[65] Gronchi A, Miah AB, Dei Tos AP, et al. Soft tissue and visceral sarcomas: ESMO-EURACAN-GENTURIS clinical practice guidelines for diagnosis, treatment and follow-up. Annals of Oncology. 2021;**32**(11):1348-1365

[66] Gamboa AC, Gronchi A, Cardona K. Soft-tissue sarcoma in adults: An update on the current state of histiotype-specific management in an era of personalized medicine. CA: A Cancer Journal for Clinicians. 2020;**70**(3):200-229

[67] Sambri A, Caldari E, Fiore M, et al. Margin assessment in soft tissue sarcomas: Review of the literature. Cancers (Basel). 2021;**13**(7):1687

[68] Kainhofer V, Smolle MA, Szkandera J, et al. The width of resection margins influences local recurrence in soft tissue sarcoma patients. European Journal of Surgical Oncology. 2016;**42**:899-906

[69] O'Donnell PW, Griffin AM, Eward WC, et al. The effect of the setting of a positive surgical margin in soft tissue sarcoma. Cancer. 2014;**120**:2866-2875

[70] Martin-Tellez KS, van Houdt WJ, van Coevorden F, et al. Isolated limb perfusion for soft tissue sarcoma: Current practices and future directions. A survey of experts and a review of literature. Cancer Treatment Reviews. 2020:102058. DOI: 10.1016/j.ctrv.2020.102058. Epub 2020 Jun 19

[71] Rosenberg SA, Baker A, Wesley R, et al. The treatment of soft-tissue sarcomas of the extremities: Prospective randomized evaluations of (1) limb-sparing surgery plus radiation therapy compared with amputation and (2) the role of adjuvant chemotherapy. Annals of Surgery. 1982;**196**(3):305-315

[72] Yang JC, Chang AE, Baker AR, et al. Randomized prospective study of the benefit of adjuvant radiation therapy in the treatment of soft tissue sarcomas of the extremity. Journal of Clinical Oncology. 1998;**16**(1):197-203

[73] Beane JD, Yang JU, White D, et al. Efficacy of adjuvant radiation therapy in the treatment of soft tissue sarcoma of the extremity: 20-year follow-up of a randomized prospective trial. Annals of Surgical Oncology. 2014;**21**(8):2484-2489

[74] Pisters PW, Harrison LB, Leung D, et al. Long-term results of a prospective randomized trial of adjuvant brachytherapy in soft tissue sarcoma. Journal of Clinical Oncology. 1996;**14**(3):859-868

[75] Alektiar B, Brennan MF, et al. Morbidity of adjuvant brachytherapy in

soft tissue sarcoma of the extremity and superficial trunk. International Journal of Radiation Oncology, Biology, Physics. 2000;**47**(5):1273-1279

[76] Koshy M, Rich SE, Mohiuddin MM. Improved survival with radiation therapy in high grade soft tissue sarcomas of the extremities: A SEER analysis. International Journal of Radiation Oncology, Biology, Physics. 2010;**77**(1):203-209

[77] Alektiar KM, Leung D, Zelefsky MJ, et al. Adjuvant radiation for stage II-B soft tissue sarcoma of the extremity. Journal of Clinical Oncology. 2002;**20**(6):1643-1650

[78] Cahlon O, Brennan MF, Jia X, et al. A postoperative nomogram for local recurrence risk in extremity soft tissue sarcomas after limb-sparing surgery without adjuvant radiation. Annals of Surgery. 2012;**255**(2):343-347

[79] Davis AM, O'Sullivan B, Bell RS, et al. Function and health status outcomes in a randomized trial comparing preoperative and postoperative radiotherapy in extremity soft tissue sarcoma. Journal of Clinical Oncology. 2002;**20**(22):4472-4477

[80] O'Sullivan B, Davis AM, Turcotte R, et al. Preoperative versus postoperative radiotherapy in soft-tissue sarcoma of the limbs: A randomised trial. The Lancet. 2002;**359**(9325):2235-2241

[81] Davis AM, O'Sullivan B, Turcotte R, et al. Late radiation morbidity following randomization to preoperative versus postoperative radiotherapy in extremity soft tissue sarcoma. Radiotherapy and Oncology. 2005;**75**(1):48-53

[82] Chung PW, Deheshi BM, Ferguson PC, et al. Radiosensitivity translates into excellent local control in extremity myxoid liposarcoma: A comparison with other soft tissue sarcomas. Cancer. 2009;**115**(14):3254-3261

[83] Alektiar KM, Velasco J, Zelefsky MJ, et al. Adjuvant radiotherapy for margin-positive high-grade soft tissue sarcoma of the extremity. International Journal of Radiation Oncology, Biology, Physics. 2000;**48**(4):1051-1058

[84] Delaney TF, Kepka L, Goldberg SI, et al. Radiation therapy for control of soft-tissue sarcomas resected with positive margins. International Journal of Radiation Oncology, Biology, Physics. 2007;**67**(5):1460-1469

[85] Tepper JE, Suit HD. Radiation therapy alone for sarcoma of soft tissue. Cancer. 1985;**56**(3):475-479

[86] Kepka L, DeLaney TF, Suit HD, et al. Results of radiation therapy for unresected soft-tissue sarcomas. International Journal of Radiation Oncology, Biology, Physics. 2005;**63**(3):852-859

[87] Alektiar KM, Leung D, Zelefsky MJ, et al. Adjuvant brachytherapy for primary high-grade soft tissue sarcoma of the extremity. Annals of Surgical Oncology. 2002;**9**(1):48-56

[88] Alektiar KM, Brennan MF, Singer S. Local control comparison of adjuvant brachytherapy to intensity-modulated radiotherapy in primary high-grade sarcoma of the extremity. Cancer. 2011;**117**(14):3229-3234

[89] Beltrami G, Rudiger HA, Mela MM, et al. Limb salvage surgery in combination with brachytherapy and external beam radiation for high-grade soft tissue sarcomas. European Journal of Surgical Oncology. 2008;**34**(7):811-816

[90] Delannes M, Thomas L, Martel P, et al. Low-dose-rate intraoperative brachytherapy combined with external beam irradiation in the conservative treatment of soft tissue sarcoma. International Journal of Radiation Oncology, Biology, Physics. 2000;**47**(1):165-169

[91] Niewald M, Fleckenstein J, Licht N, et al. Intraoperative radiotherapy (IORT) combined with external beam radiotherapy (EBRT) for soft-tissue sarcomas—A retrospective evaluation of the homburg experience in the years 1995-2007. Radiation Oncology. 2009;**4**(32)

[92] Alvegard TA, Sigurdsson H, Mouridsen H, et al. Adjuvant chemotherapy with doxorubicin in high-grade soft tissue sarcoma: A randomized trial of the Scandinavian sarcoma group. Journal of Clinical Oncology. 1989;**7**(10):1504-1513

[93] Frustaci S, Gherlinzoni F, De Paoli A, et al. Adjuvant chemotherapy for adult soft tissue sarcomas of the extremities and girdles: Results of the Italian randomized cooperative trial. Journal of Clinical Oncology. 2001;**19**(5):1238-1247

[94] Woll PJ, Reichardt P, Le Cesne A, et al. Adjuvant chemotherapy with doxorubicin, ifosfamide, and lenograstim for resected soft-tissue sarcoma (EORTC 62931): A multicentre randomised controlled trial. The Lancet Oncology. 2012;**13**(10):1045-1054

[95] Sarcoma Meta-analysis Collaboration. Adjuvant chemotherapy for localised resectable soft-tissue sarcoma of adults: Meta-analysis of individual data. The Lancet. 1997;**350**(9092):1647-1654

[96] Pervaiz N, Colterjohn N, Farrokhyar F, et al. A systematic meta-analysis of randomized controlled trials of adjuvant chemotherapy for localized resectable soft-tissue sarcoma. Cancer. 2008;**113**(3):573-581

[97] Le Cesne A, Ouali M, Leahy MG, et al. Doxorubicin-based adjuvant chemotherapy in soft tissue sarcoma: Pooled analysis of two STBSG-EORTC phase III clinical trials. Annals of Oncology. 2014;**25**(12):2425-2432

[98] Callegaro D, Miceli R, Bonval S, et al. Development and external validation of two nomograms to predict overall survival and occurrence of distant metastases in adults after surgical resection of localised soft-tissue sarcomas of the extremities: A retrospective analysis. The Lancet Oncology. 2016;**17**(5):671-680

[99] Gortzak E, Azzarelli A, Buesa J, et al. A randomised phase II study on neo-adjuvant chemotherapy for 'high-risk' adult soft-tissue sarcoma. European Journal of Cancer. 2001;**37**(9):1096-1103

[100] Palassini E, Ferrari S, Verderio P, et al. Feasibility of preoperative chemotherapy with or without radiation therapy in localized soft tissue sarcomas of limbs and superficial trunk in the Italian sarcoma group/Grupo Espanol de Investigacion en sarcomas randomized clinical trial. Journal of Clinical Oncology. 2015;**33**(31):3628-3634

[101] Gronchi A, Palmerini E, Quagliuolo V, et al. Neoadjuvant chemotherapy in high-risk soft tissue sarcomas: Final results of a randomized trial from Italian (ISG), Spanish (GEIS), French (FSG), and polish (PSG) sarcoma groups. Journal of Clinical Oncology. 2020;**38**(19):2178-2186

[102] Tanaka K, Machida R, Kawai A, et al. Results of a randomized phase

II/III study comparing perioperative adriamycin plus ifosfamide and gemcitabine plus docetaxel for high-grade soft tissue sarcomas: Japan clinical oncology group study JCOG1306. Journal of Clinical Oncology. 2020;**38**(15):11504

[103] Porter GA, Baxter NN, Pisters PW. Retroperitoneal sarcoma: A population-based analysis of epidemiology, surgery, and radiotherapy. Cancer. 2006;**106**(7):1610-1616

[104] Ecker BL, Peters MG, McMillan MT, et al. Preoperative radiotherapy in the management of retroperitoneal liposarcoma. British Journal of Surgery. 2016;**103**(13):1839-1846

[105] Nussbaum DP, Rushing CN, Lane WO, et al. Preoperative or postoperative radiotherapy versus surgery alone for retroperitoneal sarcoma:A case-control, propensity score-matched analysis of a nationwide clinical oncology database. The Lancet Oncolology. 2016;**17**(7):966-975

[106] Smith MJ, Ridgway PF, Catton CN, et al. Combined management of retroperitoneal sarcoma with dose intensification radiotherapy and resection: Long-term results of a prospective trial. Radiotherapy and Oncology. 2014;**110**(1):165-171

[107] Bonvalot S, Gronchi A, Le Péchoux C, et al. Preoperative radiotherapy plus surgery versus surgery alone for patients with primary retroperitoneal sarcoma (EORTC-62092: STRASS): A multicentre, open-label, randomised, phase 3 trial. The Lancet Oncology. 2020;**21**(10):1366-1377

[108] De Sanctis R, Giordano L, Colombo C, et al. Long-term follow-up and post-relapse outcome of patients with localized retroperitoneal sarcoma treated in the Italian sarcoma group-soft tissue sarcoma (ISG-STS) protocol 0303. Annals of Surgical Oncology. 2017;**24**(13):3872-3879

[109] Miura JT, Charlson J, Gamblin TC, et al. Impact of chemotherapy on survival in surgically resected retroperitoneal sarcoma. European Journal of Surgical Oncology. 2015;**41**(10):1386-1392

[110] Almond ML, Gronchi A, Strauss D, et al. Neoadjuvant and adjuvant strategies in retroperitoneal sarcoma. European Journal of Surgical Oncology. 2018;**44**(5):571-579

[111] Van Glabbeke M, Van Oosterom A, Oosterhuis J, et al. Prognostic factors for the outcome of chemotherapy in advanced soft tissue sarcoma: An analysis of 2185 patients treated with anthracycline-containing first-line regimens a European organization for research and treatment of cancer soft tissue and bone. Journal of Clinical Oncology. 1999;**17**:150-157

[112] O'Bryan R, Baker L, Gottlieb J, et al. Dose response evaluation of adriamycin in human neoplasia. Cancer. 1977;**39**(5):1940-1948

[113] Nielsen OS, Dombernowsky P, Mouridsen H, et al. Epirubicin is not superior to doxorubicin in the treatment of advanced soft tissue sarcomas. The perience of the EORTC soft tissue and bone sarcoma group. Sarcoma. 2000;**4**(1-2):31-35

[114] Judson I, Radford JA, Harris M, et al. Randomised phase II trial of pegylated liposomal doxorubicin versus doxorubicin in the treatment of advanced or metastatic soft tissue sarcoma: A study by the EORTC soft tissue and bone sarcoma group. European Journal of Cancer. 2001;**37**(7):870-877

[115] Ryan CW, Merimsky O, Agulnik M, et al. PICASSO III: A

phase III, placebo-controlled study of doxorubicin with or without palifosfamide in patients with metastatic soft tissue sarcoma. Journal of Clinical Oncology. 2016;**34**(32):3898-3905

[116] Edmonson J, Ryan LB, Blum R, et al. Randomized comparison of doxorubicin alone versus ifosfamide plus doxorubicin or mitomycin, doxorubicin, and cisplatin against advanced soft tissue sarcomas. Journal of Clinical Oncology. 1993;**11**(7):1269-1267

[117] Seddon B, Strauss SJ, Whelan J, et al. Gemcitabine and docetaxel versus doxorubicin as first-line treatment in previously untreated advanced unresectable or metastatic soft-tissue sarcomas (GeDDiS): A randomised controlled phase 3 trial. The Lancet Oncology. 2011;**18**(10):1397-1410

[118] Pautier P, Italiano A, Piperno-Neumann S, et al. Doxorubicin alone versus doxorubicin with trabectedin followed by trabectedin alone as first-line therapy for metastatic or unresectable leiomyosarcoma (LMS-04): A randomised, multicentre, open-label phase trial. The Lancet Oncology. 2022;**23**(8):1044-1054

[119] Stacchiotti S, Palassini E, Sanfilippo R, et al. Gemcitabine in advanced angiosarcoma: A retrospective case series analysis from the Italian rare cancer network. Annals of Oncology. 2012;**23**:501-508

[120] Pautier P, Floquet A, Penel N, et al. Randomized multicenter and stratified phase II study of gemcitabine alone versus gemcitabine and docetaxel in patients with metastatic or relapsed leiomyosarcomas: A federation Nationale des centres de Lutte Contre le (FNCLCC) French sarcoma group study. The Oncologist. 2012;**17**(9):1213-1220

[121] Le Cesne A, Blay JY, Cupissol D, et al. A randomized phase III trial comparing trabectedin to best supportive care in patients with pre-treated soft tissue sarcoma: T-SAR, a French sarcoma group trial. Annals of Oncology. 2021;**32**(8):1034-1044

[122] Schwartz GK. Trabectedin and the L-sarcomas: A decade-long odyssey. Journal of Clinical Oncology. 2015;**34**(8):769-771

[123] Schoffski P, Ray-Coquard IL, Cioffi A, et al. Activity of eribulin mesylate in patients with soft-tissue sarcoma: A phase 2 study in four independent histological subtypes. The Lancet Oncology. 2011;**12**(11):1045-1052

[124] Schöffski P, Chawla S, Maki RG, et al. Eribulin versus dacarbazine in previously treated patients with advanced liposarcoma or leiomyosarcoma: A randomised, open-label, multicentre, phase 3 trial. Lancet. 2016;**387**(10028):1629-1637

[125] Sleijfer S, Ray-Coquard I, Papai Z, et al. Pazopanib for metastatic soft-tissue sarcoma (PALETTE): A randomised, double-blind, placebo-controlled phase 3 trial. The Lancet. 2012;**379**(9829):1879-1886

[126] Van Der Graaf WT, Blay JY, Chawla SP, et al. Pazopanib, a multikinase angiogenesis inhibitor, in patients with relapsed or refractory advanced soft tissue sarcoma: A phase II study from the European organisation for research and treatment of cancer-soft tissue and bone sarcoma group (EORTC study). Journal of Clinical Oncology. 2009;**27**(19):3126-3132

[127] Valverde CM, Martin Broto J, Lopez-Martin JA, et al. Phase II clinical trial evaluating the activity and tolerability of pazopanib in patients

(pts) with advanced and/or metastatic liposarcoma (LPS): A joint Spanish sarcoma group (GEIS) and German Interdi. Journal of Clinical Oncology. 2016;**34**(15_Suppl.):11039-11039

[128] Grünwald V, Karch A, Schuler M, et al. Randomized comparison of Pazopanib and doxorubicin as first-line treatment in patients with metastatic soft tissue sarcoma age 60 years or older: Results of a German intergroup study. JCO. 2020;**38**(30). DOI: 10.1200/JCO.20.00714

[129] Tawbi HA, Burgess M, Bolejack V, et al. Pembrolizumab in advanced soft-tissue sarcoma and bone sarcoma (SARC028): A multicentre, two-cohort, single-arm, open-label, phase 2 trial. The Lancet Oncology. 2017;**18**(11):1493-1501

[130] Tawbi HA, Burgess M, Crowley J, et al. Safety and efficacy of PD-1 blockade using pembrolizumab in patients with advanced soft tissue (STS) and bone sarcomas (BS): Results of SARC028—A multicenter phase II study. Journal of Clinical Oncology. 2016;**34**(15_suppl). DOI: 10.1200/JCO.2016.34.15_suppl.11006

[131] Wilky BA, Trucco MM, Subhawong TK, et al. Axitinib plus pembrolizumab in patients with advanced sarcomas including alveolar soft-part sarcoma: A single-Centre, single-arm, phase 2 trial. The Lancet Oncology. 2019;**20**(6):837-848

[132] Martín Broto J, Le Cesne A, Reichardt P. Nirogacestat and its potential impact on desmoid tumor. Rare Tumors. 2023;**5**(15):20363613231182485. DOI: 10.1177/20363613231182485

[133] Penel N, Bui NB, Bay J, et al. Phase II trial of weekly paclitaxel for unresectable angiosarcoma: The ANGIOTAX study. Journal of Clinical Oncology. 2008;**26**(32):5269-5274

[134] Wagner AJ, Malinowska-Kolodziej I, Morgan JA, et al. Clinical activity of mTOR inhibition with sirolimus in malignant perivascular epithelioid cell tumors: Targeting the pathogenic activation of mTORC1 in tumors. Journal of Clinical Oncology. 2010;**28**(5):835

[135] Hindi N, Sanfilippo R, Stacchiotti S, et al. Systemic therapy in perivascular epithelioid cell tumors (PECOMA). Annals of Oncology. 2014;**25**(Suppl_4):iv506-iv

[136] Rutkowski P, Klimczak A, Ługowska I, et al. Long-term results of treatment of advanced dermatofibrosarcoma protuberans (DFSP) with imatinib mesylate–the impact of fibrosarcomatous transformation. European Journal of Surgical Oncology (EJSO). 2017;**43**(6):1

[137] Sirvent N, Maire G, Pedeutour F, et al. Genetics of dermatofibrosarcoma protuberans family of tumors: From ring chromosomes to tyrosine kinase inhibitor treatment. Genes, Chromosomes & Cancer. 2003;**37**(1):1-19

[138] Tejpar S, Nollet F, Li C, et al. Predominance of beta-catenin mutations and beta-catenin dysregulation in sporadic aggressive fibromatosis (desmoid tumor). Oncogene. 1999;**18**(47):6615

[139] Bulut G, Ozluk A, Erdogan AP, et al. Pazopanib: A novel treatment option for aggressive fibromatosis. Clinical Sarcoma Research. 2016;**6**(1):22

[140] Gounder MM, Lefkowitz RA, Keohan ML, et al. Activity of sorafenib against desmoid tumor/deep fibromatosis. Clinical Cancer Research. 2011;**17**(12):4082-4090

[141] de Camargo VP, Keohan ML, D'Adamo DR, et al. Clinical outcomes of systemic therapy for patients with deep fibromatosis (desmoid tumor). Cancer. 2010;**116**(9):2258-2265

[142] Constantinidou A, Jones RL, Scurr M, et al. Pegylated liposomal doxo-rubicin, an effective, well-tolerated treatment for refractory aggressive fibromatosis. European Journal of Cancer. 2009;**45**(17):2930-2934

[143] Rohail S, Fareed A, Taimuri MA, et al. Nirogacestat and its potential impact on desmoid tumor. Rare Tumors. 2023;**5**(15):20363613231182485. DOI: 10.1177/20363613231182485

[144] Tap WD, Gelderblom H, Palmerini E, et al. Pexidartinib versus placebo for advanced tenosynovial giant cell tumour (ENLIVEN): A randomised phase 3 trial. Lancet. 2019;**394**(10197):478-487

[145] Cassier PA, Gelderblom H, Stacchiotti S, et al. Efficacy of imatinib mesylate for the treatment of locally advanced and/or metastatic tenosynovial giant cell tumor/pigmented villonodular synovitis. Cancer. 2012;**118**(6):1649-1655

[146] Robinson DR, Wu Y-M, Kalyana-Sundaram S, et al. Identification of recurrent NAB2-STAT6 gene fusions in solitary fibrous tumor by integrative sequencing. Nature Genetics. 2013;**45**(2):180

[147] Maruzzo M, Martin-Liberal J, Messiou C, et al. Pazopanib as first line treatment for solitary fibrous tumours: The Royal Marsden Hospital experience. Clinical Sarcoma Research. 2015;**5**(1):5

[148] Khalifa J, Ouali M, Chaltiel L, et al. Efficacy of trabectedin in malignant solitary fibrous tumors: A retrospective analysis from the French sarcoma group. BMC Cancer. 2015;**15**(1):700

[149] Stacchiotti S, Mir O, Le Cesne A, et al. Activity of pazopanib and trabectedin in advanced alveolar soft part sarcoma. The Oncologist. 2018;**23**(1):62-70

[150] Folpe A, Deyrup A. Alveolar soft-part sarcoma: A review and update. Journal of Clinical Pathology. 2006;**59**(11):1127-1132

[151] Jakate K, Azimi F, Ali RH, et al. Endometrial sarcomas: An immunohistochemical and JAZF1 re-arrangement study in low-grade and undifferentiated tumors. Modern Pathology. 2013;**26**(1):95

[152] Yamaguchi M, Erdenebaatar C, Saito F, et al. Long-term outcome of aromatase inhibitor therapy with letrozole in patients with advanced low-grade endometrial stromal sarcoma. International Journal of Gynecological Cancer. 2015;**25**(9):1645-1651

[153] Kurman RJ, Carcangiu ML, Herrington S, et al. WHO Classification of Tumours of Female Reproductive Organs. IARC: Lyon; 2014

Chapter 2

Pre-Operative Evaluation of Soft Tissue Sarcoma

Supratim Bhattacharyya and Antarip Bhattacharya

Abstract

Soft Tissue Sarcoma (STS) is a group of heterogenous mesenchymal malignant neoplasms with variable clinical and biological behavior. Although most of the soft tissue tumors are benign in nature, a high degree of suspicion, based on clinical, radiological, cyto-histological and molecular studies, is required to diagnose STS early in its course. There are more than a hundred subtypes of STS reported in the literature. They have different prognostic implications, and often treated differently. In the last decade, owing to betterment of radiological and pathological reporting system, there has been a dramatic improvement in diagnosis and treatment of these tumors. This also led to overall improvement in awareness, and reduction in improper surgical treatment and delayed surgical referrals. However, a centralization of care is of pivotal importance for better management since STS is rare in general. The importance of multidisciplinary approach to the management of STS cannot be over emphasized. This should include a dedicated surgical team, in conjunction with radiology, pathology, radiation oncology, medical oncology, anesthesiology, physiotherapy, and nursing team. In the subsequent section we briefly discuss on the pre operative management of STS, focusing mostly on radiological and pathological evaluation.

Keywords: soft tissue sarcoma, multidisciplinary team approach, pre operative evaluation, imaging, histology, immunohistochemistry, centralization

1. Introduction

Soft Tissue Sarcomas (STS) represent a cohort of heterogenous tumors of mesenchymal cell origin (including fat, muscle, nerves, blood vessels, and other connective tissues) that account for 1% of all adult malignancies and hundreds of different histological and molecular subtypes. These different subtypes oftentimes behave differently and hence the evaluation and management of STS is diverse. And there comes the importance of Sarcoma Multidisciplinary Team (MDT) consisting of Surgical Oncologist, Orthopedician, Radiation Oncologist, Medical Oncologist, Onco-pathologist, Radiologist. The NICE guideline suggests referral to a specialist centre for any patient with a lump >5 cm, deep to fascia, fixed, immobile, painful, and increasing in size [1]. As a general rule, any indeterminate soft tissue mass is considered as STS, unless proven otherwise, and should be evaluated by Sarcoma MDT to determine the appropriate line of treatment. Owing to its rarity, evidence based management holds promising role in improving outcomes in STS. An analysis of data from 15,957 patients with STS in the National Cancer Database showed that NCCN guidelines based treatment, which largely relies on multidisciplinary approach to STS, improves survival outcomes [2]. This chapter encompasses the nuances of pre operative evaluation of STS in general.

2. Overview

Sarcomas can be broadly divided into soft tissue sarcoma and bone sarcoma. The true incidence of STS is underestimated, largely because of non inclusion of gastrointestinal stromal tumors (GIST) to the tumor registry before 2001. The anatomic site of origin has significant implications in management and prognosis of STS. The common site of origin includes extremities (43%), the trunk (10%), viscera (19%), retroperitoneum (15%), and head and neck (9%) [3]. Desmoid tumor or aggressive fibromatosis is a unique histological type associated with local invasion rather than distant metastasis. Rhabdomyosarcoma is the most common histological subtype among children and adolescents.

3. Risk factors

The evaluation of STS begins with the assessment of presence or absence of different risk factors associated with causation of STS. The risk factors are divided into modifiable and non-modifiable [4, 5].

The modifiable risk factors include

1. Prior exposure to radiation therapy

2. Chemical exposure (herbicides, such as agent orange)

The non modifiable risk factors include

Genetic syndromes as follows

Li- Fraumeni syndrome results from germline mutation of TP53 tumor suppressor gene. The syndrome results in multiple malignancies, namely STS, osteosarcoma, breast cancer, leukemia, brain tumors, adrenocortical carcinoma. The incidence of STS in this mutation ranges from 12–21% and diagnosed in early life as compared to sporadic STS [6]. Patients suspected to be suffering from this syndrome or with a known family history of this syndrome require genetic counseling prior to initiation of therapy for STS.

Familial Adenomatous Polyposis (FAP) results from germline mutation of adenomatous polyposis coli (APC) gene on chromosome 5q21. This autosomal dominant colorectal cancer syndrome is also associated with desmoid tumor (aggressive fibromatosis). The prevalence of desmoid tumor in this syndrome is much higher than that of general population [7]. The most common location of desmoid in FAP is intra-abdominal and abdominal wall (53% and 24%, respectively) which often makes surgical resection challenging. Evaluation for FAP or Gardner's syndrome is recommended for patients with desmoid tumor.

Carney- Stratakis syndrome is another autosomal dominant condition characterized by GISTs and paragangliomas. Germline loss-of-function mutations of succinate dehydrogenase (SDH) gene subunits (SDHB, SDHC, and SDHD) has been identified to be causative of this syndrome. GISTs associated with this syndrome are negative for SDHB, in contrast to GIST with KIT or PDGFRA mutations or sporadic GIST [8].

Hereditary Retinoblastoma, caused by germline mutation of RB1 tumor suppressor gene, results in higher risk of STS. Leiomyosarcoma (LMS) is reportedly the most common association, with 78% of LMS diagnosed 30 or more years after diagnosis of retinoblastoma [9].

Neurofibromatoses result from mutations in neurofibromin 1 (NF1) or neurofibromin 2 (NF2). Approximately 5% of NF patients develop STS, most commonly malignant peripheral nerve sheath tumors (MPNSTs) [10].

4. History and physical examination

Some of the STS are more common in certain age group than other. Gastrointestinal Stromal Tumor (GIST) is considered to be the most common STS in adults. Other common histological types include undifferentiated pleomorphic sarcoma (UPS), liposarcoma (LS), leiomyosarcoma (LMS), and myxofibrosarcoma (MFS). The commonest histology in children is rhabdomyosarcoma (RMS). Some of the common sarcomas of early adulthood are synovial sarcoma, alveolar soft part sarcoma, and Ewing sarcoma.

The classical history of a soft tissue sarcoma patient is a slow growing lump, increasing in size, over a period of time. Often these lumps are associated with pain. The detailed history of pain, such as rest pain, pain on activity, radiation of pain, are significant. Some tumors may show features of rapid growth which usually indicate malignant transformation or intra tumoral hemorrhage. The history of trauma, which mostly is circumstantial, is relevant as this often serves as the first point when the patient comes to know about the tumor. Also, trauma helps exclude non-malignant differentials of a lump. Change in size of the lump often indicates inflammatory masses and lymph nodes and helps excluding STS.

Physical examination should focus on estimation of the size of the mass, its location with respect to the deep fascia, its mobility and consistency. The mass should be palpated all around to determine the anatomical boundaries with respect to the compartments of the limb. Tenderness over the mass usually points towards inflammatory process. The auscultatory findings of pulsatile flow should suggest possibilities of pseudoaneurysm or vascular malformation/tumors. Sensory/motor dysfunction along the course or distal to the tumor usually indicates involvement or compression of a nerve by the tumor. A positive Tinel's sign indicates towards a nerve sheath tumor or nerve compression. A distal limb swelling may indicate venous stagnation or lymphatic obstruction. Proximal lymph nodal basins should be carefully examined to look for lymphadenopathy.

5. Imaging

Following a detailed a history to exclude presence of different risk factors and clinical examination focused on the local examination of the tumor, the next investigation to stage the disease is the imaging. Imaging plays an important role in diagnosis, guiding biopsy, pre treatment staging, surgical planning, and follow up. Although most of the STS have non specific imaging characteristics, a few histological subtypes can be diagnosed with specific imaging features of the primary and metastases.

5.1 Adipocytic tumors

i. Well Differentiated Liposarcoma (LPS) and Atypical Lipomatous Tumors (ALT)- these tumors have predilection for extremities, retroperitoneum, paratesticular and inguinal regions [11]. These tumors have predominantly fat components in imaging. Features that favor liposarcoma over lipoma include age greater than 60 years, lesion size more than 10 cm, lower extremity location, presence of thickened septations (>2 mm), nodular enhancing foci, and solid components. The sclerosing variant of well differentiated LPS are mostly seen in retroperitoneum and have predominantly non fatty components.

ii. Dedifferentiated Liposarcoma- these are mostly located in retroperitoneum, and rarely in extremities and mediastinum. It can be found in the primary well differentiated LPS or its recurrence or metastasis. They resemble undifferentiated high grade pleomorphic sarcoma and may exhibit heterogenous differentiation, such as, myogenic or osteo/chondromatous elements. On imaging, they have non fatty components, often greater than 1 cm, often showing enhancement. With the higher degree of dedifferentiation, the proportion of lipomatous component comes down progressively. Distant metastases are more common than well differentiated LPS, and mostly occur in liver and lungs.

iii. Myxoid Liposarcoma- the most common location is at the deep soft tissue of thigh. They tend to occur in young to middle aged adults. On imaging, they have a well circumscribed, multilobulated, septated appearance. The myxoid component takes very high signal intensity in T2 weighted MRI, with heterogenous enhancement pattern. The high grade tumors usually show more than 10 cm size, deep location, lack of lobulations, and more than 5% fatty component [12, 13]. Myxoid LPS has a tendency to metastasize to extrapulmonary sites, especially to paraspinal region, intramuscular fat pad, bone, retroperitoneum, and the opposite extremity. Whole body MRI is an useful tool for screening of bony and soft tissue metastasis in myxoid LPS.

iv. Pleomorphic Liposarcoma- these are the least common subtype of LPS and tend to occur in elderly patients, specially in deep soft tissue of the extremities. They have a high propensity for early metastasis and have a poor prognosis. The imaging usually shows features of aggressive sarcoma with evidence of local invasion having little fat component.

5.2 Fibroblastic/myofibroblastic tumors

i. Dermatofibrosarcoma Protuberans- this rare form comprises of 6% of all STS. They are more common in men and in fourth and fifth decade. They have t(17;22) translocation, resulting in platelet derived growth factor receptor activation. The most common site of occurrence is the trunk. In 20% cases there is fibrosarcomatous transformation [14]. The typical MRI findings include a lobular or nodular enhancing intermediate signal intensity lesion with focal protuberance. T2 hyperintensity is noted in myxoid lesions. Hemorrhage and necrosis indicates fibrosarcomatous transformation.

ii. Myxofibrosarcoma- it is more common after sixth decade and extremity is the most common location (75%). Most are subcutaneous tumors. Because of myxoid components, they are typically hyper enhancing in T2 weighted MRI. Often there are septations, necrosis, and hemorrhage. T2 hypointense pseudocapsules may be present. A characteristic feature is unencapsulated margin and infiltrative growth pattern along the fascial planes, and this explains the high risk of local recurrence post resection. This infiltrative nature is visible on MRI as a high signal 'tail sign' that discriminates this tumor from other myxoid neoplasms.

5.3 Smooth muscle tumors

Leiomyosarcoma (LMS): they account for about 9% of STS. The commonest sites of involvement are uterus, retroperitoneum. They are the most common sarcoma of large blood vessels. On MRI, they show non specific features, such as T1 iso-intensity with moderate hyper intensity in T2. Hemorrhage, necrosis, cystic changes are common for larger tumors [15]. They often show features of calcification and ossification.

5.4 Skeletal muscle tumors

Rhabdomyosarcoma (RMS): it is the most common STS of childhood. In children, the most common site of affection is head and neck parameningeal region, while in adults the commonest site of involvement is extremities followed by genitourinary system. There are three histological subtypes. The commonest one is embryonal type (50%) occurring in the first decade of life, and affects head and neck and genitourinary system. The alveolar type (30%) has more preponderance to affect the trunk and extremities of adolescents. They also tend to affect the lymph nodes. The pleomorphic subtype is common in adults more than 45 years and commonly affect lower extremities. Embryonal RMS usually presents with poorly circumscribed heterogenous mass with moderately high signal intensity in T2 weighted images [16]. The botryoid type is characterized by multiple ring enhancing regions inside the mass. There may be features of infiltration to the surrounding bones. Alveolar RMS present as infiltrative heterogenous mass with area of necrosis. They show moderately high signal intensity in T2 images. The pleomorphic type shows marked high signal intensity in T2 images with features of infiltration.

5.5 Vascular tumors

Angiosarcoma: the majority of angiosarcoma are subcutaneous in origin, with less than 25% arising from deep soft tissue. Factors increasing the risk of angiosarcoma include chronic lymphedema, radiation exposure, familial syndromes (e.g., neurofibromatosis type 1, Klippel-Trenaunay-Weber syndrome), and implants. These are tumors with very aggressive biology with high potential for locoregional and distant metastases. MR signal characteristics include intermediate on T1 and heterogeneously high on T2 images. Areas of high signal on T1 usually suggests intra tumoral hemorrhage. Deeper tumors may show flow void, but this is typically absent in subcutaneous tumors.

5.6 Nerve sheath tumors

These include benign tumors, such as schwannoma and neurofibroma, and malignant tumors, such as Malignant Peripheral Nerve Sheath Tumors (MPNST).

MPNSTs may arise de novo, or in the background of benign neurofibromas in the setting on NF1. MPNSTs account for about 5–10% of all STS and occur in fourth to sixth decade of life with equal sex predilection, except for those arising in the background of NF1 where it appears early in life and more common in male (about 80%) [17]. Some MPNSTs have rhabdomyoblastic components inside the tumor and are classified as malignant triton tumor, which manifest an aggressive course and poorer outcome. The most common nerves involved are sciatic nerve, brachial plexus, and sacral plexus. These tumors show non specific imaging features like intermediate signal intensity on T1 and iso to high signal on T2 weighted images. They often share imaging characteristics of benign neurogenic tumors such as fusiform appearance around an involved nerve, split fat sign, bright rim sign, fascicular sign, and atrophy of the supplying muscle owing to denervation. Clinical pictures such as high growth rate, size more than 5 cm, infiltrative margin favor the diagnosis of malignant tumor more than benign. Imaging features indicative of malignancy are heterogeneous high signal on T1, irregular peripheral enhancement pattern, and peritumoral edema [18].

5.7 Tumors of uncertain differentiation

i. Synovial Sarcoma (SS): these account for 5–10% of STS and usually manifest in young adults. They are pathologically classified as monophasic (spindle cell component), biphasic (spindle cell and epithelial components), and poorly differentiated subtypes. The t(X;18) translocation is characteristic and seen in 95% of the tumors. The most common site of origin is extremity, especially around the knee and adjoining tendon sheath. On imaging, SS are septated multilobulated mass with heterogenous signal intensity on T1 and T2 images, due to cystic changes, necrosis, hemorrhage, calcification. They may demonstrate 'fluid- fluid levels' due to layering hemorrhage, and 'bowl of grapes' due to T2 hyperintense lobulations on the background of hypointense septa [19]. Aggressive tumors show signs of invasion to bone and infiltration of adjacent organs. They have a very rate of lung metastasis as well as lymph nodal metastasis.

ii. Alveolar Soft Part Sarcoma (APSS): these rare tumors are usually seen in children and young adults, and tend to occur more in lower extremities. Owing to highly vascular nature, they often present as pulsatile mass with audible bruits. On imaging, they appear as well circumscribed lobulated masses with moderately high signal intensity on T1 and T2 images and marked contrast enhancement. They often have internal signal voids due to intra tumoral vessels [20]. Most present with lung metastasis at diagnosis. Other sites of metastasis include lymph nodes, bones, and brain. Despite having an aggressive biology, they susually have a good survival.

iii. Extraskeletal Ewing Sarcoma (EES): they belong to the Ewing Sarcoma (ES) family of tumors, that include ES, EES, Primitive Neuroectodermal Tumors (PNET), and Askin tumor. ES belongs to small round blue cell tumor family, arising from neuroectodermal cells, with classical t(11;22) translocation. They arise mostly from deep soft tissue of extremities, retroperitoneum, chest wall, and paravertebral regions (most commonly in cervical and sacral spinal level). On imaging, they have a bulky heterogenous appearance with adjacent organ invasion. They are hypo or iso intense to the skeletal muscle on T1 and heterogeneously hyperintense on T2 images, with frequent occurrence of central necrosis [21]. The most common sites of metastasis include lungs, lymph nodes, and bones.

iv. Extraskeletal Osteosarcoma (EO): they are very rare and very aggressive. They tend to occur in post radiation setting, in fifth decade and later. The commonest site of involvement is thigh, followed by upper extremity, retroperitoneum and trunk. The MRI findings include well circumscribed, inhomogeneous mass on T1 and T2, with or without heterogeneous contrast enhancement and often with pseudocapsule formation. Mineralization is seen n 50–70% cases, and may cause signal void [22]. Aggressive tumors may have intra tumoral hemorrhage, necrosis. They have a high propensity for metastasis and poor overall survival.

v. Aggressive Angiomyxoma: they are rare locally aggressive tumors most commonly arising from perineum and lower pelvis. They often present late due to displacement of adjacent organs without symptoms. Owing to myxoid matrix, they are T2 hyper intense. The presence of fibrovascular stroma leads to swirling or laminated appearance [23].

vi. Desmoplastic Small Round Cell Tumor: these rare tumors arise from peritoneal layers of younger adults, more commonly in male. They belong to the family of small round blue cell tumors. The common imaging appearance include bulky, heterogenous peritoneum based masses, without distinct site of origin. The pelvis and paravesical regions are frequent sites of affection. Ascites is common.

vii. Solitary Fibrous Tumor (SFT): these rare tumors appear in middle aged individuals without sex predilection. Histological hallmark of these tumors are CD34 positivity (seen in 80–100% cases) and over expression of STAT6 protein. The commonest site of origin is the pleura and about 20% cases are malignant. The extra-pleural tumors usually originate from retroperitoneum, pelvis, proximal extremity, and abdominal wall. On MRI, these are well circumscribed, lobular masses and having inhomogeneous signal intensity on T2 images. The fibrous and hemorrhagic component gives a T2 hypo intensity while the myxoid and cystic component gives T2 hyper intensity images.

viii. Gastrointestinal Stromal Tumor (GIST): GISTs are the most common mesenchymal tumors originating from GI tract. They are believed to grow from the intestinal cell of Kajal. Pathologically they are characterized by activating mutation of tyrosine kinase receptors, namely c-kit (CD117)or platelet derived growth factor alpha. On imaging, GISTs present as predominantly exophytic soft tissue masses arising from the bowel wall with variable areas of hemorrhage and necrosis [24]. The most common site of origin is stomach. Metastasis is mostly limited to liver and peritoneum, however lymph nodal metastasis is noted in succinate dehydrogenase deficient GISTs.

6. Biopsy

The treatment of soft tissue sarcoma is dependent on the histological type and hence the importance of a correct biopsy cannot be over emphasized. The goal of biopsy is to provide adequate tissue for histology and immunohistochemistry. Furthermore, the biopsy tract is often the place for seedling of cancer cells, so the biopsy should always be planned in a way so that the biopsy site and the biopsy tract can be taken out with the tumor during definitive resection.

Soft tissue sarcomas (STS) comprise of neoplasia arising from soft tissues which are mostly uncommon tumors of diverse histology, different biology and varied outcomes. Recent advancements in the field of pathology with the advent of immunohistochemistry (IHC), cytogenetics and molecular genetics have caused change in the classification and diagnosis of STS. It has also changed the clinical management and prognosis of these tumors.

The WHO classification of STS considers the clinical, histological and genetic factors and it divides STS into four categories viz. benign, intermediate (locally aggressive), intermediate (metastasizing) and malignant [25, 26].

The benign tumors usually do not recur while the intermediate (locally aggressive) tumors tend to recur locally and follow an infiltrative destructive growth pattern. However, they usually lack the potential to metastasize. On the other hand, the intermediate (metastasizing) tumors in addition to being locally aggressive, have the ability to metastasize in few cases, the risk of it being <2% and is cannot be predicted by its histomorphology. Malignant soft tissue tumors show a significant ability of distant metastasis, which ranges from 20% to almost 100% depending on the histological type and grade [26, 27].

Biopsy of STS is done by either of open or closed approach. While an open biopsy usually requires an operating room for obtaining tissue, a closed biopsy is usually an out patient procedure that relies on taking tissue using core biopsy needle with or without image guidance.

A blind biopsy without image guidance is usually the choice for superficial mass which are easily palpable and the most representative area (solid part of a heterogenous mass) is easily accessible to the clinician obtaining biopsy. The mass must always be away from any critical underlying structure to prevent inadvertent injury. In all other cases an image guided biopsy would be justified over a blind technique.

Close biopsies are associated with less morbidity, but the yield of tissue is less. It can be in the form of fine needle aspiration cytology (FNAC) or core needle biopsy (CNB). FNAC has limited use in STS due to the fact that it gives only small sample of cells from the tumor and often it is not possible to run extended batteries of stains and cytogenetics to determine the accurate subtype.

Core needle biopsy (CNB), on the other hand, provides pathologist enough tissue sample to determine the exact histopathological subtype. Also it provides adequate material for immunohistochemistry and cytogenetics.

Irrespective of the biopsy technique employed, the biopsy track must always be planned in a way to incorporate during the surgical resection of the mass. Also, the biopsy track must not contaminate multiple compartments, joint spaces, and neurovascular structures.

Open biopsies are divided into incisional and excisional biopsy. Although excisional biopsy is generally not recommended for STS, incisional biopsy provides sufficient tissue for subtyping STS and has the advantage of immediate frozen section analysis to confirm the presence of representative tissue. An open biopsy incision should be planned after consultation with the primary surgeon who subsequently operates on the patient. The wound must be closed after securing proper hemostasis to prevent formation of post operative hematoma which would otherwise contaminate the adjacent tissue planes unnecessarily.

6.1 Grading

The two predominant grading systems for STS are the Fédération Nationale des Centres de Lutte Contre le Cancer (FNCLCC) and the National Cancer Institute (NCI) systems [28, 29]. Each of these systems consists of three grades, which rely on factors such as mitotic activity, necrosis, and differentiation. The NCI system additionally takes into account cellularity and pleomorphism for specific subtypes of sarcoma. The grading system correlates to the prognosis of the disease. The TNM staging recommends the FNCLCC system for classification into 'high grade' and 'low grade' [30, 31]. The FNCLCC grading system is shown in **Table 1**.

6.2 Morphological categories

Apart from grading, histopathological examination of STS also includes architectural pattern, the appearance of the cells and the stromal characteristics. This creates several different categories which are classified based on morphological features as well as immunohistochemical markers. The classification is as demonstrated in **Table 2**.

Histological classification and diagnosis of STS is quite complex. It is sometimes difficult to precisely classify the tumor based on fine needle aspiration (FNA) and

Tumor differentiation	
Score 1	Sarcomas closely resembling normal adult mesenchymal tissue (e.g. well differentiated liposarcoma and leiomyosarcoma)
Score 2	Sarcomas for which histological typing is certain (e.g. myxoid liposarcoma & conventional leiomyosarcoma)
Score 3	Embryonal and undifferential sarcomas, Pleomorphic sarcomas, synovial sarcomas, osteosarcomas, PNET)
Mitotic count	
Score 1	0–9 mitoses per HPF
Score 2	10–19 mitoses per HPF
Score 3	> = 20 mitoses per HPF
Tumor necrosis	
Score 0	No tumor necrosis
Score 1	Less than or equal to 50% tumor necrosis
Score 2	More than 50% tumor necrosis
Histological grade	
Grade 1	Total score 2, 3
Grade 2	Total score 4, 5
Grade 3	Total score 6, 7, 8

Table 1.
Histological grading according to FNCLCC.

Morphological category	IHC parameters
Fascicular spindle cell sarcomas	
Fibrosarcoma	Vimentin
Leiomyosarcoma	SMA, HHF 35, Calponin, Desmin ±
Spindle cell RMS	Desmin+, Myogenin+
Synovial sarcoma	S-100±, EMA+
MPNST	S-100+, EMA–
Solitary fibrous tumor	CD34+, CD99–, CD31–
Myxoid Soft Tissue Sarcomas	
Myxoid liposarcoma	MDM2+,CD34±, novel IHC antibody to the TLS/EWS-CHOP chimeric oncoproteins
Myxoid chondrosarcoma	Vim+, Synaptophysin±, EMA±
Myxoid DFSP	CD34
Myxoid MFH (myxofibrosarcoma)	CD34+, HMGA1 and HMGA2
Botryoid Embryonal RMS	Desmin, Myogenin
Myxoid leiomyosarcoma	SMA, HHF 35, Desmin, Myogenin
Epitheloid Soft Tissue Sarcomas	
Alveolar soft part sarcoma	Desmin, SMA
Epithelioid sarcoma	CK, EMA, Vimentin, CD34±
Epithelioid angiosarcoma	CD31, Factor VIII, CD34, FLI-1
Epithelioid haemangioendothelioma	CD31, Factor VIII, CD34, FLI-1
Extra gastrointestinal stromal tumor	CD117, CD34±
Malignant Rhabdoid tumor	Polyphenotypic, Loss of INI1 protein
Malignant mesothelioma	Calretinin, Thrombomodulin
Synovial sarcoma	EMA, Cytokeratin, S100±
Sclerosing epithelioid fibrosarcoma	Vimentin
Clear cell sarcoma	HMB45, Melan1 *EWSR1-ATF* fusion
Round Cell Soft Tissue Sarcomas	
Alveolar RMS	Desmin, Myogenin
Desmoplastic small round cell tumor of childhood	Polyphenotypic
Embryonal RMS	Desmin, Myogenin
Extra skeletal ES/PNET	CD99, FLI-1
Round cell liposarcoma	S-100
Small cell osteosarcoma	Vimentin
Malignant hemangiopericytoma	CD34
Pleomorphic Sarcomas	
Pleomorphic undifferentiated sarcoma	Vimentin
Malignant fibrous histiocytoma	Alpha 1 antitrypsin, alpha-1-antichymotrypsin
Pleomorphic liposarcoma	MDM2 and CDK4

Morphological category	IHC parameters
Pleomorphic RMS	Desmin, Myogenin
Pleomorphic MPNST	S100
Pleomorphic leiomyosarcoma	SMA, SMA, Desmin
Pleomorphic angiosarcoma	CD31, Factor VIII, CD34, FLI-1
Chondro-Osseous STS	
Mesenchymal Chondrosarcoma	S-100
Extra skeletal osteosarcoma	Vimentin
Clear Cell Lesions	
Clear cell sarcoma of soft tissue	S-100, HMB45, NSE, CD57, *EWSR1-ATF* fusion gene
Clear cell myomelanocytic tumor	HMB45, MelanA±, SMA±

Table 2.
Morphological categories of STS.

core biopsy specimens. The role of frozen section intraoperatively is also limited and only provides information about the margin status and that tumor tissue has been obtained.

In certain cases, a few reactive processes may mimic sarcomas. The distinction with reactive cells is made on the fact that the latter usually does not demonstrate any atypical mitosis or nuclear atypia which is characteristic of a neoplastic cell. The reactive cells have large vesicular nuclei, prominent nucleoli and basophilic cytoplasm.

In terms of grading, histopathological information obtained by small biopsies (FNA/core needle) can sometimes be inaccurate. This may cause a high-grade lesion being diagnosed as low grade because features like necrosis may be missed. Thus, proper classification is sometimes only possible on open excision biopsies or resected specimens. Grading of STS also becomes unreliable if chemotherapy or radiotherapy has been administered prior to biopsy.

6.3 Immunohistochemistry

Immunohistochemical staining has played a pivotal role in enhancing the precision of STS diagnosis, especially given that several histologic subtypes exhibit distinct chromosome translocations and gene rearrangements.

Some of them include Ewing's sarcoma, t(11,22); synovial sarcoma, t(X,18); myxoid liposarcoma, t(12,16); and clear cell sarcoma, t(12,22) [32].

The primary approach in immunohistochemistry (IHC) involves two key steps: first, the exclusion of non-mesenchymal tumors, and second, the determination of the cell lineage of any identified mesenchymal tumors. This process necessitates the use of a panel of diverse immunostains rather than relying on a single marker to minimize the risk of misdiagnosis due to unusual antigen expression, such as cytokeratin in angiosarcoma [33]. Employing a predefined and thoughtfully selected small panel based on distinct patterns is recommended, as it offers a more efficient and cost-effective approach. The initial selection of IHC markers should consistently include a broad keratin (pancytokeratin), S100, and vimentin. A positive keratin result suggests a primary carcinoma, while a positive S100 stain should trigger the application of additional melanoma markers. Leukocyte common antigen (LCA) and CD30

STS type	Fusion gene	Chromosomal location	Clinical significance
Ewing sarcoma	EWSR1-FLI1	22q12.2 11q24.3	Most common fusion gene in Ewing sarcoma.
Alveolar rhabdomyosarcoma	PAX3-FOXO1 or PAX7-FOXO1	2q36.1 1p36.13 13q14.11	Found in most cases of alveolar rhabdomyosarcoma.
Synovial sarcoma	SS18-SSX1 or SS18-SSX2	18q11.2 X chr X chr	Specific translocation seen in synovial sarcoma.
Myxoid liposarcoma	FUS-DDIT3	16p11.2 12q13.12	Characteristic fusion gene in myxoid liposarcoma.
Dermatofibrosarcoma protuberans	COL1A1-PDGFB	17q21.33 22q13.1	Common fusion gene in dermatofibrosarcoma protuberans.
Clear cell sarcoma	EWSR1-ATF1	22q12.2 12q13.2	Associated with clear cell sarcoma of soft tissue.
Desmoplastic small round cell tumor	EWSR1-WT1	22q12.2 11p13	Identifying fusion gene in desmoplastic small round cell tumor.
Infantile fibrosarcoma	ETV6-NTRK3	12p13.2 15q25.3	Occurs in infantile fibrosarcoma cases.
Inflammatory myofibroblastic tumor	ALK	2p23	ALK gene rearrangements in this tumor type.

Table 3.
STS with fusion genes.

are pivotal markers for distinguishing Hodgkin's lymphomas, large cell lymphomas (including anaplastic large cell lymphoma), and follicular dendritic cell tumors [33].

A unique soft tissue sarcoma showing both epithelial and mesenchymal differentiation is synovial sarcoma. IHC is useful in the diagnosis and to distinguish the monophasic spindle cell from the other sarcomas. Cytokeratins and EMA are strongly positive in most cases and is usually co-expressed with vimentin. CD34 is positive in around 50% cases. A strong CD99 membrane positivity is usually seen in most Ewing's sarcoma/Primitive Neuroectodermal Tumors, though it tends to be more sensitive than specific [34].

Though histopathology and immunohistochemistry can diagnose a majority of soft tissue sarcomas, it is to be noted that the results should be considered in the context of all available data since there is a tendency of aberrant antigen expression in soft-tissue tumors. There are a variety of pitfalls in the diagnosis of STS including technical factors and there is even an estimate that IHC adds confusion to the diagnostic process in 5–10% cases [35].

6.4 Detection of fusion genes

The detection of fusion genes in soft tissue sarcomas typically involves various laboratory techniques and tests (**Table 3**). Here are some common methods for detecting fusion genes:

1. Fluorescence In Situ Hybridization (FISH): FISH is a molecular cytogenetic technique that uses fluorescent probes to detect specific DNA sequences. It can

identify chromosomal rearrangements that result in fusion genes. This method is commonly used in clinical diagnostics for detecting fusion genes in soft tissue sarcomas.

2. Reverse Transcription Polymerase Chain Reaction (RT-PCR): RT-PCR is a molecular biology technique that allows for the amplification and detection of RNA molecules. It is commonly used to detect fusion transcripts in sarcomas. Specific primers designed for the known fusion gene breakpoints are used to amplify and identify the fusion transcript.

3. Next-Generation Sequencing (NGS): NGS is a high-throughput sequencing technology that can identify fusion genes by sequencing the entire genome or transcriptome. This approach is particularly useful for discovering novel or rare fusion events and provides comprehensive genomic information.

4. Immunohistochemistry (IHC): In some cases, immunohistochemistry can indirectly suggest the presence of fusion genes. Specific antibodies can target fusion protein products or surrogate markers associated with fusion genes, aiding in diagnosis.

5. Cytogenetic Analysis: Traditional cytogenetic techniques, such as karyotyping and G-banding, can reveal chromosomal abnormalities that may indicate the presence of fusion genes. These methods are particularly valuable for detecting large chromosomal rearrangements.

6. RNA Sequencing: RNA sequencing can provide valuable information about the transcriptome, including the presence of fusion transcripts. It is especially useful for discovering new fusion events and understanding the functional consequences of fusion genes.

7. Array Comparative Genomic Hybridization (aCGH): aCGH can detect genomic imbalances, including chromosomal gains or losses, which may be indicative of fusion genes in some cases.

The choice of detection method often depends on the specific fusion gene of interest, the available resources, and the laboratory's expertise. A combination of these techniques may be used to accurately identify fusion genes in soft tissue sarcomas, aiding in both diagnosis and potential targeted therapy decisions.

7. Predictive nomograms

Despite curative intent treatment of STS, approximately 25% of patients develop metastatic disease in long run [36]. The incidence reaches 50% for those with high risk tumors (size >5 cm, location deep to deep fascia, high grade histology) [37, 38]. The ability to predict recurrence and survival in long run help us make the treatment planning more rational. It also makes the patient more compliant with the treatment decision making. Therefore, prognostic nomograms incorporating clinical parameters such as tumor site, size, histological pattern, grade, patient age, performance status, are useful tool for treatment decision making, patient counseling, meeting patient's expectations, post treatment follow up strategy making, and also for conducting clinical trials. The first nomogram introduced for STS was from the Memorial Sloan Kettering Cancer Center (MSKCC) group and is widely known as MSKCC Sarcoma Nomogram. It incorporated five covariates, including age at diagnosis, tumor size, histological subtype, histological grade, and anatomical site. It was aimed at determining 12-year sarcoma specific death probability for low and high grade tumors.

In 2003, the MSKCC group produced another nomogram to predict 5-year sarcoma specific death probability for locally recurrent disease based on the same covariates. Later it was understood that the anatomical site plays a major role in predicting prognosis of sarcoma, and hence several site specific nomograms were introduced to predict locoregional recurrence, disease free survival (DFS), and overall survival (OS). Anaya et al. described a nomogram which took histology, completeness of resection, age, multifocality, tumor size, and presentation as covariates [39]. In a nomogram described by Ardiono et al., histology, FNCLCC grade, size, surgical resection margin, and age were taken as covariates [40]. Tan et al. described another nomogram which included histology, extent of resection, number of organs resected, size, and radiation [41]. In 2013, Gronchi et al. described a nomogram studying more than 500 patients [42]. This nomogram was externally validated and endorsed by the American Joint Committee on Cancer (AJCC) staging system for retroperitoneal sarcoma. This nomogram included FNCLCC grade, tumor size, histology, age, multifocality, and extent of surgical resection into account. This predicts 7 year OS for different histological subtypes, including dedifferentiated liposarcoma, leiomyosarcoma, malignant peripheral nerve sheath tumor, solitary fibrous tumor, undifferentiated pleomorphic sarcoma, well differentiated liposarcoma etc.

One of the major limitations of using nomograms is that they predict the survival based on post operative findings, and hence the ability to determine the pre operative prediction of survival is limited.

8. Centralization of care

Soft tissue sarcoma has more than a hundred histological and molecular subtypes. They often behave differently from one another. And the heterogeneity is not just confined to diagnosis, but also in treatment decision making and prognosticating the disease. It is a proven fact that the outcome over short and long term is better for institutes dedicated to treatment of similar malignancies. The treatment decision is entirely based on multidisciplinary approach, which necessarily includes surgical oncologist, orthopedic oncologist, radiation oncologist, medical oncologist, dedicated radiologist and pathologist, physiotherapist, rehabilitation therapist, and dedicated nursing team. There are studies to support the better short term as well as long term outcomes when the patients of STS are treated in high volume centers having a dedicated sarcoma team. Keung et al. reported in their study of more than a thousand retroperitoneal sarcoma cases that patients treated at high-volume centers had lower 30-day readmission, lower 30-day and 90-day mortality, and longer median and 5-year overall survival [43]. These findings were similar to a French study of over thirty-five thousand patients showing that those treated at specialized sarcoma referral centers had a low risk of local relapse, progression, and death (hazard ratio [HR], 0.64, 0.83, and 0.68, respectively; all $P < .001$) [44, 45]. Also the centralisation of care would enable us to perform multi-institutional studies to answer the unmet needs in the management of STS which ultimately benefits the patients. We live in the era of personalized cancer care, and treatment of STS has undergone a paradigm shift in a decade time, fundamentally based on the same ideation.

9. Conclusion

STS accounts for 1% of all malignancies. Hence, having a robust data on management strategy is a difficult task. However, with the advancement of different treatment modalities, there has been a paradigm shift in the management of these tumors. The sarcoma specific centers having multidisciplinary approach to personalized cancer care for STS is definitely the way forward. Continued collaborative efforts from these centers will allow future studies sufficiently powered to generate further evidence and betterment of STS specific treatment.

Conflict of interest

The authors declare no conflict of interest.

Author details

Supratim Bhattacharyya* and Antarip Bhattacharya
Apollo Multispecialty Hospital and Apollo Cancer Centre, Kolkata, India

*Address all correspondence to: dr.supratimb@gmail.com

References

[1] Grimer R, Athanasou N, Gerrand C, Judson I, Lewis I, Morland B, et al. UK guidelines for the management of bone sarcomas. Sarcoma. 2010;**2010**:317462. DOI: 10.1155/2010/317462

[2] Voss RK, Chiang YJ, Torres KE, et al. Adherence to National Comprehensive Cancer Network Guidelines is associated with improved survival for patients with stage 2A and stages 2B and 3 extremity and superficial trunk soft tissue sarcoma. Annals of Surgical Oncology. 2017;**24**:3271-3278. DOI: 10.1245/s10434-017-6015-z

[3] Pisters PWT, Weiss M, Maki R. Soft-tissue sarcomas. In: Haller DG, Wagman LD, Camphausen C, et al., editors. Cancer Management: A Multidisciplinary Approach Medical, Surgical, & Radiation Oncology. 14th ed. UBM Medica Healthcare Publications LLC; 2011

[4] Brady MS, Gaynor JJ, Brennan MF. Radiation-associated sarcoma of bone and soft tissue. Archives of Surgery. 1992;**127**(12):1379-1385. DOI: 10.1001/archsurg.1992.01420120013002

[5] Penel N, Grosjean J, Robin YM, Vanseymortier L, Clisant S, Adenis A. Frequency of certain established risk factors in soft tissue sarcomas in adults: A prospective descriptive study of 658 cases. Sarcoma. 2008;**2008**:459386. DOI: 10.1155/2008/459386

[6] Olivier M, Goldgar DE, Sodha N, Ohgaki H, Kleihues P, Hainaut P, et al. Li-Fraumeni and related syndromes: Correlation between tumor type, family structure, and TP53 genotype. Cancer Research. 2003;**63**(20):6643-6650

[7] Nieuwenhuis MH, Lefevre JH, Bülow S, Järvinen H, Bertario L, Kernéis S, et al. Family history, surgery, and APC mutation are risk factors for desmoid tumors in familial adenomatous polyposis: An international cohort study. Diseases of the Colon and Rectum. 2011;**54**(10):1229-1234. DOI: 10.1097/DCR.0b013e318227e4e8

[8] Gill AJ, Chou A, Vilain R, Clarkson A, Lui M, Jin R, et al. Immunohistochemistry for SDHB divides gastrointestinal stromal tumors (GISTs) into 2 distinct types. The American Journal of Surgical Pathology. 2010;**34**(5):636-644. DOI: 10.1097/PAS.0b013e3181d6150d

[9] Kleinerman RA, Tucker MA, Abramson DH, Seddon JM, Tarone RE, Fraumeni JF Jr. Risk of soft tissue sarcomas by individual subtype in survivors of hereditary retinoblastoma. Journal of the National Cancer Institute. 2007;**99**(1):24-31. DOI: 10.1093/jnci/djk002

[10] Brems H, Beert E, de Ravel T, Legius E. Mechanisms in the pathogenesis of malignant tumours in neurofibromatosis type 1. The Lancet Oncology. 2009;**10**(5):508-515. DOI: 10.1016/S1470-2045(09)70033-6

[11] Brisson M, Kashima T, Delaney D, Tirabosco R, Clarke A, Cro S, et al. MRI characteristics of lipoma and atypical lipomatous tumor/well-differentiated liposarcoma: Retrospective comparison with histology and MDM2 gene amplification. Skeletal Radiology. 2013;**42**(5):635-647. DOI: 10.1007/s00256-012-1517-z

[12] Tateishi U, Hasegawa T, Beppu Y, Kawai A, Satake M, Moriyama N. Prognostic significance of MRI findings in patients with myxoid-round cell

liposarcoma. AJR. American Journal of Roentgenology. 2004;**182**(3):725-731. DOI: 10.2214/ajr.182.3.1820725

[13] Löwenthal D, Zeile M, Niederhagen M, Fehlberg S, Schnapauff D, Pink D, et al. Differentiation of myxoid liposarcoma by magnetic resonance imaging: A histopathologic correlation. Acta Radiologica. 2014;**55**(8):952-960. DOI: 10.1177/0284185113508114

[14] Hoesly PM, Lowe GC, Lohse CM, Brewer JD, Lehman JS. Prognostic impact of fibrosarcomatous transformation in dermatofibrosarcoma protuberans: A cohort study. Journal of the American Academy of Dermatology. 2015;**72**(3):419-425. DOI: 10.1016/j.jaad.2014.11.020

[15] Hartman DS, Hayes WS, Choyke PL, Tibbetts GP. From the archives of the AFIP. Leiomyosarcoma of the retroperitoneum and inferior vena cava: Radiologic-pathologic correlation. Radiographics. 1992;**12**(6):1203-1220. DOI: 10.1148/radiographics.12.6.1439022

[16] Allen SD, Moskovic EC, Fisher C, Thomas JM. Adult rhabdomyosarcoma: Cross-sectional imaging findings including histopathologic correlation. AJR. American Journal of Roentgenology. 2007;**189**(2):371-377. DOI: 10.2214/AJR.07.2065

[17] Murphey MD, Smith WS, Smith SE, Kransdorf MJ, Temple HT. From the archives of the AFIP. Imaging of musculoskeletal neurogenic tumors: Radiologic-pathologic correlation. Radiographics. 1999;**19**(5):1253-1280. DOI: 10.1148/radiographics.19.5.g99se101253

[18] Zhang Z, Deng L, Ding L, Meng Q. MR imaging differentiation of malignant soft tissue tumors from peripheral schwannomas with large size and heterogeneous signal intensity. European Journal of Radiology. 2015;**84**(5):940-946. DOI: 10.1016/j.ejrad.2015.02.003

[19] Murphey MD, Gibson MS, Jennings BT, Crespo-Rodríguez AM, Fanburg-Smith J, Gajewski DA. From the archives of the AFIP: Imaging of synovial sarcoma with radiologic-pathologic correlation. Radiographics. 2006;**26**(5):1543-1565. DOI: 10.1148/rg.265065084

[20] Suh JS, Cho J, Lee SH, Shin KH, Yang WI, Lee JH, et al. Alveolar soft part sarcoma: MR and angiographic findings. Skeletal Radiology. 2000;**29**(12):680-689. DOI: 10.1007/s002560000285

[21] Murphey MD, Senchak LT, Mambalam PK, Logie CI, Klassen-Fischer MK, Kransdorf MJ. From the radiologic pathology archives: Ewing sarcoma family of tumors: Radiologic-pathologic correlation. Radiographics. 2013;**33**(3):803-831. DOI: 10.1148/rg.333135005

[22] Mc Auley G, Jagannathan J, O'Regan K, Krajewski KM, Hornick JL, Butrynski J, et al. Extraskeletal osteosarcoma: Spectrum of imaging findings. AJR. American Journal of Roentgenology. 2012;**198**(1):W31-W37. DOI: 10.2214/AJR.11.6927

[23] Srinivasan S, Krishnan V, Ali SZ, et al. "Swirl sign" of aggressive angiomyxoma-a lesser known diagnostic sign. Clinical Imaging. 2014;**38**(5):751-754. DOI: 10.12998/wjcc.v6.i14.811

[24] Tirumani SH, Jagannathan JP, Krajewski KM, Shinagare AB, Jacene H, Ramaiya NH. Imatinib and beyond in gastrointestinal stromal tumors: A radiologist's perspective. AJR. American Journal of Roentgenology. 2013;**201**(4):801-810. DOI: 10.2214/AJR.12.10003

[25] Hogendoom PCW, Collin F, Daugaard S, et al. Changing concepts in the pathological basis of soft tissue and bone sarcoma tumor. European Journal of Cancer. 2004;**40**:1644-1654. DOI: 10.1016/j.ejca.2004.04.004

[26] Fletcher CDM, Unni KK, Mertens F. WHO Classification of Tumors. Pathology and Genetics of Tumors of Soft Tissue and Bone. Lyon: IARC Press; 2002

[27] Fletcher CD. The evolving classification of soft tissue tumours: An update based on the new WHO classification. Histopathology. 2006;**48**(1):3-12. DOI: 10.1111/j.1365-2559.2005.02284.x

[28] Guillou L, Coindre JM, Bonichon F, Nguyen BB, Terrier P, Collin F, et al. Comparative study of the National Cancer Institute and French Federation of Cancer Centers Sarcoma Group grading systems in a population of 410 adult patients with soft tissue sarcoma. Journal of Clinical Oncology. 1997;**15**(1):350-362. DOI: 10.1200/JCO.1997.15.1.350

[29] Coindre JM, Trojani M, Contesso G, et al. Reproducibility of a histopathologic grading system for adult soft tissue sarcoma. Cancer. 1986;**58**(2):306-309. DOI: 10.1002/1097-0142(19860715)58:2<306

[30] Edge SB, Compton CC. The American joint committee on Cancer: The 7th edition of the AJCC cancer staging manual and the future of TNM. Annals of Surgical Oncology. 2010;**17**(6):1471-1474. DOI: 10.1245/s10434-010-0985-4

[31] Sobin LH, Gospodarowicz M, Wittekind C. UICC TNM Classification of Malignant Tumours. 7th ed. New York, NY: Wiley-Liss; in press, NLM ID: 101511218 [Book]

[32] Fletcher CDM, Bridge JA, Hogendoorn PC, et al., editors. WHO Classification of Tumors of Soft Tissue and Bone. 4th ed. Lyon, France: IARC Press; 2013

[33] Folpe AL, Cooper K. Best practices in diagnostic immunohistochemistry: Pleomorphic cutaneous spindle cell tumors. Archives of Pathology & Laboratory Medicine. 2007;**131**(10):1517-1524. DOI: 10.5858/2007-131-1517-BPIDIP

[34] Fujimura Y, Ohno T, Siddique H, Lee L, Rao VN, Reddy ES. The EWS-ATF-1 gene involved in malignant melanoma of soft parts with t(12;22) chromosome translocation, encodes a constitutive transcriptional activator. Oncogene. 1996;**12**(1):159-167

[35] Brooks JS. Immunohistochemistry in the differential diagnosis of soft tissue tumors. Monographs in Pathology. 1996;**38**:65-128

[36] Lindberg RD, Martin RG, Romsdahl MM, Barkley HT Jr. Conservative surgery and postoperative radiotherapy in 300 adults with soft-tissue sarcomas. Cancer. 1981;**47**(10):2391-2397. DOI: 10.1002/1097-0142(19810515)47:10<2391::aid-cncr2820471012>3.0.co;2-b

[37] Markhede G, Angervall L, Stener B. A multivariate analysis of the prognosis after surgical treatment of malignant soft-tissue tumors. Cancer. 1982;**49**(8):1721-1733. DOI: 10.1002/1097-0142(19820415)49:8<1721::aid-cncr2820490832>3.0.co;2-x

[38] Mandard AM, Petiot JF, Marnay J, Mandard JC, Chasle J, de Ranieri E, et al. Prognostic factors in soft tissue sarcomas. A multivariate analysis of 109 cases. Cancer. 1989;**63**(7):1437-1451.

DOI: 10.1002/1097-0142 (19890401)63:7<1437::aid-cncr2820630735>3.0.co;2-q

[39] Anaya DA, Lahat G, Wang X, Xiao L, Pisters PW, Cormier JN, et al. Postoperative nomogram for survival of patients with retroperitoneal sarcoma treated with curative intent. Annals of Oncology. 2010;**21**(2):397-402. DOI: 10.1093/annonc/mdp298

[40] Ardoino I, Miceli R, Berselli M, Mariani L, Biganzoli E, Fiore M, et al. Histology-specific nomogram for primary retroperitoneal soft tissue sarcoma. Cancer. 2010;**116**(10):2429-2436. DOI: 10.1002/cncr.25057

[41] Tan MC, Brennan MF, Kuk D, Agaram NP, Antonescu CR, Qin LX, et al. Histology-based classification predicts pattern of recurrence and improves risk stratification in primary retroperitoneal sarcoma. Annals of Surgery. 2016;**263**(3):593-600. DOI: 10.1097/SLA.0000000000001149. PMID: 25915910

[42] Gronchi A, Miceli R, Shurell E, Eilber FC, Eilber FR, Anaya DA, et al. Outcome prediction in primary resected retroperitoneal soft tissue sarcoma: Histology-specific overall survival and disease-free survival nomograms built on major sarcoma center data sets. Journal of Clinical Oncology. 2013;**31**(13):1649-1655. DOI: 10.1200/JCO.2012.44.3747

[43] Brooks JS. Immunohistochemistry in the differential diagnosis of soft tissue tumors. Monographs in Pathology. 1996;**38**:65-128

[44] Keung EZ, Chiang YJ, Cormier JN, Torres KE, Hunt KK, Feig BW, et al. Treatment at low-volume hospitals is associated with reduced short-term and long-term outcomes for patients with retroperitoneal sarcoma. Cancer. 2018;**124**(23):4495-4503. DOI: 10.1002/cncr.31699

[45] Blay JY, Honoré C, Stoeckle E, Meeus P, Jafari M, Gouin F, et al. Surgery in reference centers improves survival of sarcoma patients: A nationwide study. Annals of Oncology. 2019;**30**(7):1143-1153. DOI: 10.1093/annonc/mdz124 Erratum in: Annals of Oncology 2019 Jun 05

Chapter 3

Thoracic Follicular Dendritic Cell Sarcoma

Vinay V. and Priya Sharma

Abstract

Follicular dendritic cell sarcoma (FDCS), which makes up 0.4% of all soft tissue sarcomas, is an uncommon low-grade malignant tumor that develops from follicular dendritic cells in germinal centres of lymphoid tissue. The pathophysiology of FDCS is unknown. It can arise in both nodal and extra-nodal areas harboring FDCs and is commonly diagnosed in middle-aged individual who are in their fifth decade of life. The extranodal lymph node locations include the liver, spleen, and GI tract, where FDCS occurs most frequently (79.4%). It is quite uncommon to develop a pulmonary follicular dendritic cell sarcoma. At the microscopic scale, the FDCS displays a wide range of architectural patterns, including fascicular, storiform, whorled, and diffuse patterns. It is frequently not considered a differential diagnosis for a spindle cell neoplasm because of its rarity, misdiagnosis, and diagnostic difficulties. There is no effective treatment for this uncommon tumor, and the value of adjuvant therapy is still debatable. The median survival period following surgery for thoracic FDCS is approximately 4.41 years, with a 5-year recurrence-free survival rate of 47%. Patients diagnosed with localized disease exhibit a 5-year overall survival rate of 55%, whereas those with metastatic disease have a lower rate of 38%.

Keywords: follicular dendritic cell, follicular dendritic cell sarcoma, extranodal spread, pulmonary involvement, immunohistochemistry, outcome

1. Introduction

Tumors related to macrophage/monocyte and dendritic cell morphologies are collectively referred to as histiocytic neoplasms. They include both benign (e.g., Erdheim-Chester illness, Langerhans cell histiocytosis/LCH) and neoplastic (interdigitating dendritic cell sarcoma, histiocytic sarcomas, indeterminate cell sarcomas, FDCS, Langerhans cell sarcoma) conditions [1, 2]. FDCS, a unique and distinctive low-grade sarcoma showing spindle-shaped cells grouped in a whorled pattern, usually manifests as a slowly growing asymptomatic mass. Numerous examples have been reported to date since Monda and Rosai first identified primary malignant neoplasms (PMN) that had traits of follicular dendritic cells (FDC) in 1986 [3]. Perez-Ordonez and Rosai's 1998 publication was the first in-depth analysis of FDC tumors [4]. Among the lymph node groups, the most affected ones include cervical, axillary, mediastinal, and intra-abdominal sites, whereas the lung, spleen, and liver are the most affected extranodal sites [5, 6]. Although once thought to be a low-grade malignancy, FDCS shows a significant malignant potential. At least, 40% of cases have local recurrence and 25% of cases have metastatic spread. Because of the short follow-up durations in numerous researches in the literature, even these numbers are an understatement [7]. However, due to their rarity compared to spindle cell sarcoma or carcinoma, spindle cell tumors do not necessarily raise concerns for FDCS when they appear as extranodal neoplasms. Moreover, the extensive variety of morphological features in FDCS poses a greater challenge in its diagnosis. It is worth noting that the reported misdiagnosis rate for FDCS in extranodal sites can be as high as 58%, affirming the idea that cases of FDCS have likely remained undetected [8].

2. Epidemiology

Follicular dendritic cell sarcoma (FDCS) is an exceptionally uncommon tumor, and its occurrence within the thoracic region is even rarer. Nevertheless, the precise incidence remains undetermined [9]. Literature consists of a few cases, less than 50 (**Table 1**). FDCS comprise <0.4% of soft tissue sarcomas. In a meta-analysis of 462 FDCS cases, the median age (range = 8–90 years) of occurrence was fifth decade of life with no gender predilection [6]. FDCS's unusual and distinctive inflammatory pseudotumor-like variant tends to affect women more than other FDCS variants [25]. The fact that several cases have been documented from East Asia raises the idea that FDCS may be more common among some ethnic groups or regions [6].

3. Pathogenesis

3.1 Origin and function of FDCs

Follicular dendritic cells, also known as dendritic reticulum cells, is a vital component in B-cell follicles. Their primary function is to gather, hold, and deliver antigens to nearby B cells. They are present in lymphoid follicles both primary and secondary [26], and their origin is mesenchymal [27]. Follicular dendritic cells were initially described as 'embryonal non-phagocytic reticulum cell' in Maximow's 1927 illustration of B follicles in human lymph nodes [28]. Under electron microscopy, FDCs exhibited interdigitations and extension of their plasma membranes, closely interacting with other germinal centre cells. This shows their potential significance in the germinal centre response, which has now been proven by a wide range of experiments [29]. Within the immune system, histiocytic and dendritic cells play a vital role by aiding in phagocytosis, processing antigens, and presenting these antigens to B and T cells. FDCs are nonlymphoid, nonphagocytic immune system accessory cells that are crucial for antigen presentation and controlling germinal centre reactivity [7, 30–32]. They create a dense network inside lymphoid follicles.

A key function of the FDC is luring B and T cells to B follicles through the secretion of CXCL13 (C-X-C chemokine motif ligand 13) and the interaction with B cells through integrins and their appropriate receptors. Immunocomplexes that are 'exposed' to germinal centre B-cells border the FDC cell membrane. By releasing numerous B-cell growth factors, mainly B activating factor (BAFF), FDC helps B cells survive and mature. During the germinal centre reaction, FDC plays a role in the apoptosis and phagocytosis of B cells with low-affinity B-cell receptors, a process

Sl no	Authors	Type of Report	Site of FDCs	Age (years)	Gender	Clinical Presentation	Treatment given	Outcome
1	Fassina et al. [10]	Case report	Mediastinal mass	48	Male	Chest pain	NA	NA
2	Shah et al. [11]	Case report	Left lung mass	33	Male	Dry cough	NA	NA
3	Leipsic et al. [12]	Case report	Middle Mediastinum	43	Male	Chest Pain	NA	NA
4	Dening et al. [13]	Case report	Right lower lobe nodule	64	Female	Cough and breathlessness	NA	NA
5	Bushan et al. [14]	Case report	Anterosuperior mediastinal mass	34	Male	Fever and malaise	Surgery followed by chemoradiation	No recurrence at 6 months Follow up.
6	Lee et al. [15]	Case report	Posterior mediastinum	63	Male	Dry cough, breathlessness	Surgery	NA
7	Butler et al. [16]	Case report	Right main bronchus lesion	19	Female	Cough, fever, dyspnoea	Surgery with lymphadenectomy	No recurrence at 2 years Follow up
8	Wang et al. [17]	Case report	Lung parenchyma	76	Female	Dyspnoea	Surgery	Expired
9	Miyoshi et al. [18]	Case report	Posterior Mediastinum	16	Female	Incidental finding	Surgery	No recurrence at 2 years Follow up
10	Ulises et al. [19]	Case report	Posterior mediastinum	59	Male	Oral ulcers/ pemphigus	Complete excision with 1 cycle of Cyclophosphamide, Doxorubicin, Vincristine, and Prednisone.	No recurrence at 2 months Follow up
11	Xu et al. [20]	Case report	Right lateral chest wall	44	Male	Chest wall pain	Tumor resection with lymphadenectomy of level I axillary nodes.	No recurrence at 18 months Follow up.
12	Ilonen et al. [21]	Case report	Posterior Mediastinum	57	Male	Incidental finding	Chemotherapy (Doxorubicin, Ifosfamide, Mesna), Surgery, Radiotherapy	No recurrence at 2 years Follow up
13	He et al. [22]	Case report	Right lower lobe mass	64	Female	Incidental finding	Surgery	No recurrence at 6 months follow-up
14	Li et al. [23]	Case report	Right hila of Lung	29	Male	Cough, expectoration	Surgery Tacrolimus Cyclosporine	Symptomatic improvement at 1 month
15	Vinay et al. [24]	Case report	Left upper lobe mass	34	Male	Chest Pain	Surgery	NA

Table 1.
Summary of extranodal follicular dendritic cell sarcomas reported in the thorax (according to year of publication).

mediated by Mfge8 produced by FDC [33]. FDCs can impact the adaptive immune response by recognizing environmental innate stimuli, such as microbial lipopolysaccharides, through Toll-like receptor 4 (TLR4). This recognition triggers TLR signaling, which in turn, promotes the synthesis of proteins such as CXCL13, TGF-1, and BAFF that contribute to B cell survival, recruitment, and class-switch recombination (**Figure 1**) [34].

Inflammatory pseudotumor-like fibroblastic/follicular dendritic cell neoplasm is an uncommon neoplasm that arises from dendritic cells. Within the World Health Organization (WHO) classification of hematological and lymphoid organ cancers, sarcoma is recognized as a unique entity. There are unique clinical characteristics of this tumor, including a predilection for young to middle-aged women, an occurrence

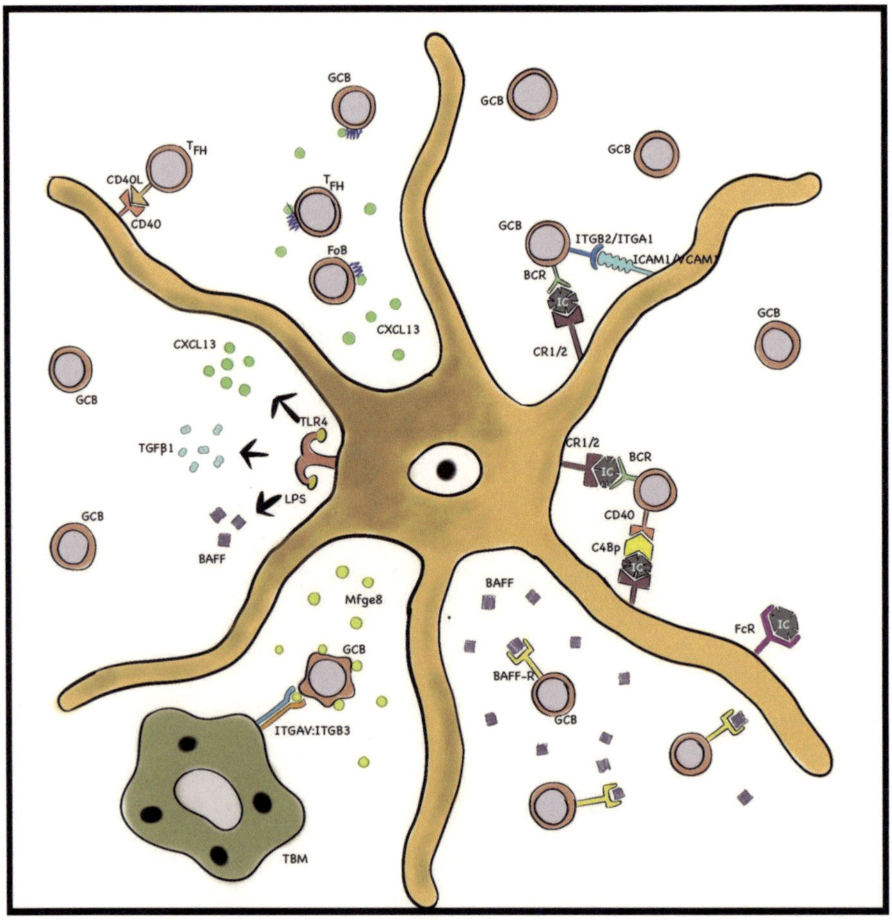

Figure 1.
By secreting CXCL13 (C-X-C motif chemokine ligand 13) and connecting with B cells via cognate receptors and integrins, FDC plays a critical role in attracting T and B cells to B follicles. Immunocomplexes that are 'exposed' to germinal Centre B cells border the FDC cell membrane. FDC promotes B-cell survival and maturation by releasing a number of B-cell growth factors, including BAFF (B-activating factor). The germinal Centre response, which is mediated by Mfge8 generated by FDC, results in the apoptosis and phagocytization of B-cells with low-affinity B-cell receptors. FDC can influence the acquired response by detecting, through TLR-4 (toll-like receptor 4), ambient innate stimuli (such as microbial lipopolysaccharides), which leads to TLR signaling that stimulates the synthesis of proteins (CXCL13, TGF-1, and BAFF) and promote B cell survival, recruitment, and class-switch recombination.

in the liver or spleen, and the presence of Epstein-Barr virus (EBV) positive neoplastic cells [35]. This could be explained by EBV entering these cells due to FDCs expressing CD21, which functions as a receptor for the virus. Additionally, FDCs have been linked to myasthenia gravis, paraneoplastic pemphigus, and Castleman disease. Epidermal growth factor receptor is expressed in FDCS and non-neoplastic FDCs of Castleman disease, which may encourage the persistence of FDCs and allow for mutations that could lead to FDCS [6, 36].

3.2 Morphology of FDC

Long dendritiform processes and an abundance of poorly defined eosinophilic cytoplasm are characteristics of FDC. The nuclear membrane is clearly defined, the chromatin is finely scattered, and the nucleus is big, ovoid to spherical in shape with a tiny eosinophilic nucleolus. Typically, bi- or multinucleated FDC exhibit a 'kissing' pattern of nuclear molding and overlap [37]; these characteristics make it easier to identify FDC in cytological smears. On electron microscopy, the FDC's cytoplasmic extensions are coated in an amorphous substance that resembles immunocomplexes and form a complex network connected by desmosomes [38]. Various FDC markers, including CD21 (C3d receptor), CD23, CD35 (C3b receptor), R4/23, DRC-1 (R4/25), CNA.42, Ki-M4p, Ki-M4, and Ki-FDC1p, effectively highlight the dendritic characteristics of FDCs on both frozen and paraffin sections. Compared to other malignant histiocytic tumors, FDCS exhibits a unique immunophenotype.

The mechanism of acquiring neoplastic potential by these FDCs is still not well studied, and more research in this is needed. As such, no universal driver translocation or mutation has been identified by comprehensive genomic investigation. A wide range of chromosomal instability, dysregulation of cell cycle progression, activation of nuclear factor kappa beta (NF-kB), mitogen-activated protein kinase (MAPK), and broad immunological evasion are also related to FDCS [39, 40]. BRAF V600E mutations, present in many histiocytic diseases and are affecting 20% of people with FDCS, might be more prevalent in the inflammatory form [41]. Epstein-Barr virus is regularly linked to the inflammatory version [42], while human herpesvirus 8 (HHV-8) is not known to be involved [43].

Association with mutations in TP53, PTEN, and NF-kB pathways has been noted in the literature [40, 44]. The expression of PD-L1 and PD-L2 and copy number increases at 9p24 implying immune surveillance escape may be involved in tumor development [40]. EZH2 was found to be overexpressed in FDCS tumors in 67% of cases, whereas p-ERK1/2 (phospho-extracellular signal-related protein kinases 1 and 2) were robustly expressed in 80% of cases [45]. Notably, nearly all FDCS cases have elevated levels of the epidermal growth factor receptor (EGFR), a hallmark of epithelial malignancies. The survival and expansion of FDCS cells may depend on EGFR signaling, which is triggered by ligands in the microenvironment [46].

4. Clinical presentation

FDCS does not have a gender predilection. It primarily occurs in adults, typically appearing at a median age of 49 years ranging from 8 to 90 years. There have been very few reported instances of this condition in pediatric patients [6]. FDCS has the potential to affect various anatomical regions. A higher frequency of involvement is seen in extranodal sites (79.4%), particularly in the liver, spleen, gastrointestinal tract, tonsil/adenoid, mediastinum, and lungs compared to nodal involvement (15%) [38]. FDCS frequently appears as a gradually developing mass that can either be symptom-free or accompanied by discomfort. The variant resembling an inflammatory pseudotumor (IPT) displays distinctive clinical attributes. Females are more likely to be impacted, as is the existence of EBV infection inside the tumor cells with the involvement of the liver or spleen and frequent systemic symptoms such as fever, malaise, and weight loss [22, 42, 47–51]. FDCS is found to be associated with many conditions such as paraneoplastic pemphigus with or without myasthenia gravis [52–56], lymphoproliferative conditions such as Castleman Disease-Hyaline vascular type (HV-CD) [57] and Sjogren's syndrome [58] manifesting predominantly in extranodal sites. FDCS is also observed in conjunction with neoplasms such as lymphomas, leukemias, and malignant neoplasms of epithelial or melanocytic origin [38].

5. Differential diagnosis

Because of histopathological diversity and the potential to manifest at various locations, FDCS can be mistaken for various types of tumors and even inflammatory processes. The reported rates of misidentification range from 30 to 58% especially when it arises from extranodal sites [59, 60]. It might be mistaken with interdigitating dendritic cell sarcoma (IDCS), Langerhans cell histiocytosis (LCH), Kaposi sarcoma, spindle cell thymoma, metastatic melanoma, metastatic carcinoma, inflammatory myofibroblastic tumor, pleomorphic sarcoma, solitary fibrous tumor, and gastrointestinal stromal tumor (GIST).

IDCSs are uncommon tumors believed to originate from interdigitating dendritic cells within the nodal paracortex. They are typically found in lymph nodes or the spleen and are associated with an aggressive nature. Histologically indistinguishable from FDCS, IDCS generally displays a higher level of atypical features and lacks the bundled structures and spiral growth pattern commonly observed in most cases of FDCS that necessitates immunohistochemical studies for a definite diagnosis. IDCS is positive for S100, negative or focally positive for clusterin. LCH comprises oval-shaped Langerhans cells, characterized by their nuclei exhibiting grooves, folds, or indentations. These nuclei have fine chromatin, inconspicuous nucleoli, and thin nuclear membranes. The cells possess moderately abundant cytoplasm that appears slightly eosinophilic. Langerhans cells are typically positive for CD1a and langerin. In the case of Kaposi's sarcoma, the condition is characterized by atypical spindle-shaped cells that form slit-like vascular spaces containing red blood cells. Immunohistochemistry (IHC) reveals the presence of positive cells for HHV8.

Spindle cell thymoma is commonly located in the anterior mediastinum. It is characterized by the presence of spindle-shaped cells exhibiting a growth pattern that ranges from fascicular to whorls. These spindle cells test positive for keratin (AE1/AE3). In metastatic carcinoma, the epithelioid cells are found in sheets, clusters, or as single cell with pronounced nuclear atypia. These cells also show positivity for keratin (AE1/AE3). Metastatic melanoma exhibits varying cytology, which may include epithelioid or spindle-shaped cells displaying nuclear atypia and prominent nucleoli. Additionally, the cytoplasm of these cells may contain brown pigment (melanin). IHC in metastatic melanoma shows positivity for S100 and MelanA. Inflammatory myofibroblastic tumor (IMT) comprises spindled myofibroblasts and fibroblasts with bland nuclei. IMT cells are positive for anaplastic lymphoma kinase-1 (ALK1).

Pleomorphic sarcoma is composed of pleomorphic cells that exhibit a diverse range of cytological characteristics, which can encompass spindled, plasmacytoid, epithelioid, or multinucleated forms. Notably, this type of sarcoma does not demonstrate positivity for clusterin, CXCL13, CD21, CD23, and CD35. Positivity for DOG1 and STAT6 are seen in solitary fibrous tumors that are usually negative in FDCS [61, 62]. In FDCS, tumor markers CD34 and CD117, typically used to identify gastrointestinal stromal tumors (GIST) tend to show negative results [38, 62].

6. Diagnosis

6.1 Histopathology

Macroscopically, FDCS appears as a gray-yellow firm mass with a well-circumscribed surface. Necrosis can be visible in few areas. This tumor has occasionally been confused with lymphoma, mesenchymal tumors such as gastrointestinal stromal tumors or solitary fibrous tumors, or poorly differentiated carcinoma, depending on the site of its presentation. The diagnosis of FDCS is consistently confirmed through immunohistochemistry, and it often requires the use of multiple FDC markers because the loss of antigens is a common occurrence [37]. Limited studies have described the EBV-associated FDCS. Based on the number and growth pattern of EBV, the degree of lymphoplasmacytic infiltration, and characteristics of the intratumoral blood vessels, the tumors were classified into the following groups: classic type (53.8%), lymphoma-like subtype (38.5%), and hemangioma-like subtype (7.7%) [63].

Most FDCSs are considered low-grade sarcomas. Histological sections reveal a spindle cell proliferation exhibiting diverse architectural arrangements with the most common being storiform or whorled (reminiscent of meningiomas) bundles (**Figure 2A** and **B**), fascicles (**Figure 2C** and **D**), trabecular formations, or widespread sheets. Multiple growth patterns are frequently observable within the same tumor. Abundant lymphocytes are often dispersed throughout the tumor, occupying the spaces between tumor cells and the areas around blood vessels. Some cases exhibit a predominance of B-cell lymphocytes, whereas others feature a preponderance of T-cell lymphocytes. Occasional multinucleated cells, albeit in small quantities, may be present, resembling Warthin-Finkeldey giant cells. These cells typically exhibit indistinct boundaries, resulting in a syncytial appearance. Their cytoplasm is moderately abundant, with a pale eosinophilic hue and the possibility of having a fibrillary texture. Tumor cells typically feature elongated or ovoid nuclei characterized by a thin nuclear membrane, vesicular or granular chromatin, and small nucleoli (**Figure 2E** and **F**). Nuclear pseudoinclusions are sporadically observed, and their frequency may increase following radiation therapy. The mitotic rate is generally low, ranging from 0 to 10 mitoses per 10 high-power fields, and necrosis is infrequently detected. The proliferation index, typically represented by Ki-67, typically falls within the range of 1–25% (**Figure 3D**). This index can be elevated in cases demonstrating clear atypia [63]. As lymphocytes, including both B and T cells as well as plasma cells, are often commingled with tumor cells in IPT-like variants, recognizing tumor cells can be challenging [38]. The histological features of this disorder may include prominent nuclear atypia, including irregular nuclear membranes and hyperchromatic nuclei, and high mitotic counts ranging from 11 to 35 mitoses per 10 high-power field. Additionally, extensive necrosis may be present. These high-grade features are

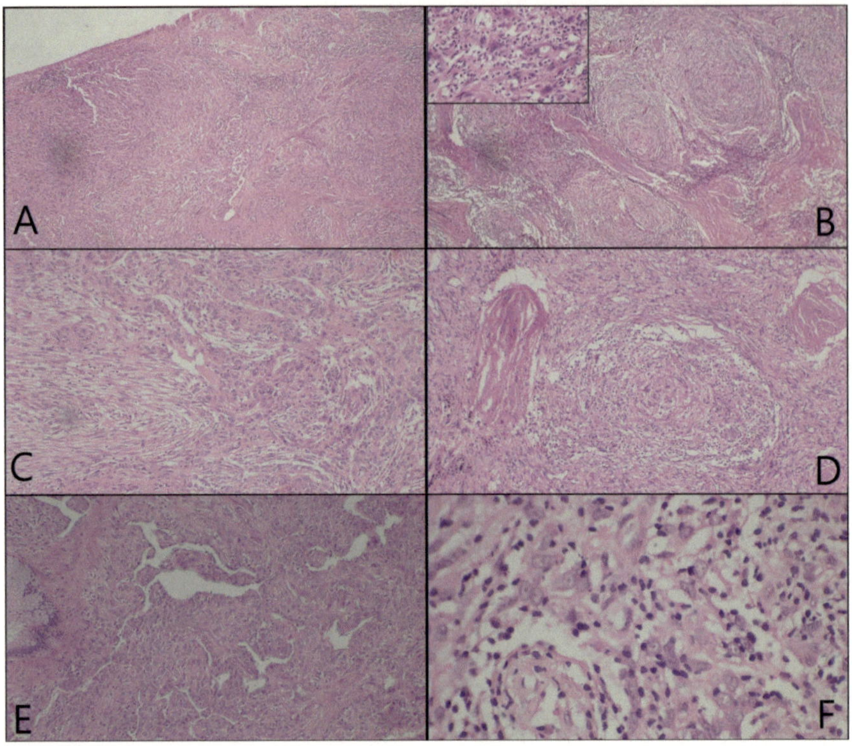

Figure 2.
Histological sections display a cellular arrangement featuring elongated to spindle-shaped cells with eosinophilic nuclei, interspersed among lymphocytes, eosinophils, and plasma cells (Image 2A & B). The spindle cells are arranged in irregular bundles, and the cytoplasm appears pale or eosinophilic, with nuclei exhibiting moderate cytoplasmic cells organized in fascicles [40× (Image 2C & 2D), 100× (Image 2E & 2F)].

typically linked to lesions located in deeper tissue layers and are indicative of a higher likelihood of recurrence or metastasis [62].

6.2 Immunophenotype

Diagnosing FDCS typically necessitates support from immunohistochemistry, and the utilization of multiple FDC markers is often imperative due to the frequent occurrence of antigen loss. Tumor cells exhibit varying degrees of positivity for CD21 (as shown in **Figure 3A** and **B**) and CD23, as well as CD35. In contrast, clusterin, podoplanin (**Figure 3C**), and CXCL13 consistently display higher expression levels, demonstrating high specificity in distinguishing them from tumors that may resemble FDCS. As a marker for FDCS, podoplanin (D2-40) exhibits high sensitivity and strong membrane staining [62]. EGFR expression is frequently detected in FDCS, although its specificity is relatively limited. Reports indicate that FDCS may exhibit positive staining for epithelial membrane antigen, CD68, S-100 protein, and, albeit rarely, cytokeratin and CD20 [37]. On occasion, reports have indicated reactivity in FDCS for S100, smooth muscle actin, CD68, and EMA. FDCS usually yields negative results in tests for CD1a, langerin, CD34 (**Figure 3E**), CD45 (**Figure 3F**), lysozyme, CD163, myeloperoxidase, CD3, CD79a, cytokeratin, MART1, and HMB45 [38]. In recent advancements, FDC-secreted protein (FDCSP), SSTR2A, and serglycin (SRGN) have surfaced as valuable markers for the purpose of identification [64].

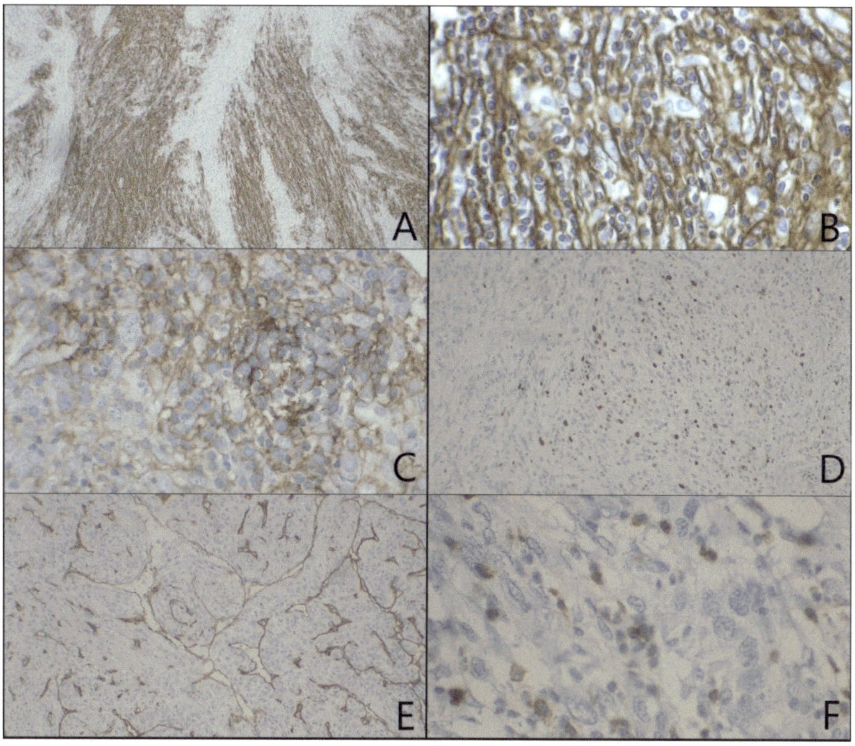

Figure 3.
FDCS cells showing IHC positivity to CD 21 (Image 3A & 3B), podoplanin (Image 3C), and Ki-67 (Image 3D). Negative for CD 34 (Image 3E) and CD 45 (Image 3F).

6.3 Electron microscopy

In the realm of electron microscopy, characteristic diagnostic elements in FDCS consists of elongated and intricately interlocking cytoplasmic extensions, occasionally forming a maze-like configuration, as well as desmosome-like connections, whereas cytoplasm typically exhibits limited organelles, notably lacking Birbeck granules and lysosomes [62].

7. Genetics and molecular findings

Vermi and colleagues in their FDCS series examined the prevalent genetic variations in EGFR (specifically substitutions in exons 18 and 21, as well as deletion of exon 19), KRAS (exon 1), NRAS (exons 1 and 2), and PI3KCA (exons 9 and 20). Notably, no mutations in these genes were detected in any of the cases studied. In an FDCS cell line, the EGFR pathway was activated, showing that local cognate ligands are involved, rather than oncogenic mutations [46]. Genomic alterations found in FDCS includes single nucleotide variations, loss/deletions, amplification of genes, copy number gains, and fusion rearrangements [39]. Five unique translocations leading to fusion proteins were identified in four cases: MAP3K1-GCOM1, NTRK1-PDIA3, TYK2-ATPAF2, HDGRFP3-SHC4, and BPTF-WDR72 [38]. FDCS is distinguished by genetic modifications affecting genes within the NF-κB regulatory pathway, encompassing copy number loss or missense mutations in TRAF3, SOCS3, TNFAIP3, and NFKBIA [65]. Additionally, mutated cell-cycle regulators leading to recurrent homozygous deletions of tumor suppressor genes CDKN2A, RB1, and CYLD and BIRC3 has also been observed [39]. Go et al. employed direct Sanger sequencing and peptide nucleic acid clamp quantitative polymerase chain reaction to ascertain the presence of mutations and detected BRAFV600E mutation in 18.5% (5 out of 27) of FDCS cases [41]. PDGFRB N666S mutation occurring in HV-CD was found in FDCS patients with history of Castleman disease. While PD-L1 expression is frequently observed in FDCS, a substantial number of cases within a comprehensive dataset exhibited a low mutational burden, measuring less than six mutations per mega base [65]. This discovery raises doubts about the potential effectiveness of immunotherapy as a treatment approach for this neoplasm [38].

8. Treatment

Various approaches have been addressed such as surgery, chemotherapy, tyrosine kinase inhibitors, and radiotherapy because FDCS lacks specific treatment guidelines. Surgery remains the mainstay of treatment in FDCS patients with localized disease. Systemic therapies used in the metastatic setting include doxorubicin, ifosfamide, or gemcitabine-based regimens, which provided prolonged stable disease [66]. Numerous regimens incorporating gemcitabine have been experimented. The rate of complete responders was 42% for those undergoing gemcitabine combined with taxotere therapy, as reported by Jain et al. [67]. In contrast, gemcitabine and taxane therapy achieved an impressive 80% complete response rate, with a notable median response duration of 13.4 months in docetaxel combination therapy, as highlighted by Conry et al. [68]. Various systemic treatment protocols have been explored, encompassing doxorubicin and ifosfamide; vincristine, doxorubicin, and cyclophosphamide (VAC); ifosfamide and etoposide with or without carboplatin (ICE/IE); cyclophosphamide, doxorubicin, vincristine, and prednisone; as well as gemcitabine, either alone or in combination with docetaxel, carboplatin, and irinotecan. A number of patients received tyrosine kinase inhibitors, including sorafenib, sirolimus, ridaforolimus, sunitinib, brivanib, imatinib, cabozantinib, and pazopanib, which resulted in extended positive outcomes, both when administered as a first-line treatment or in subsequent therapy. Research indicates that the maturation and activation of dendritic cells were impeded by vascular endothelial growth factor (VEGF). However, this inhibitory effect was counteracted using VEGF inhibitors, including bevacizumab, sorafenib, and sunitinib [69]. Enhanced comprehension of the molecular characteristics and causative factors behind this tumor could pave the way for innovative therapeutic approaches.

9. Outcome

The pooled analysis of published case reports indicated that patients who were administered adjuvant radiotherapy (RT; 51 in total) did not experience improved overall survival (OS) when compared to those who underwent surgery alone (78 in total) [6]. In FDCS, pleomorphism or prominent nuclear atypia, a size of 6 cm or more, five or more mitoses per 10 high-power fields, and coagulative necrosis on microscopy are associated with an unfavorable prognosis [70]. In the study conducted by Saygin et al., they documented 2-year survival rates of 82% for early-stage cases, 80% for locally infiltrated tumors, and 42% for cases with distant metastasis [6]. In the study conducted by Gounder M et al., it was observed that the median overall survival (OS) exhibited significance difference among patients with localized disease (9.8 years), in contrast to individuals with metastatic or recurrent disease (2.69 years). Median survival in thoracic FDCS was 4.41 years, and the 5-year overall survival was 0.47. Local recurrence or metastasis has been observed in one-third of the diagnosed FDCS cases. The 5-year survival rate for individuals diagnosed with localized disease is 55%, while it drops to 38% for those with metastatic disease [66].

10. Conclusions

The thoracic extranodal FDCS will probably continue to be an underappreciated tumor. Thoracic FDCs contains several characteristic histological features that should serve as an indication to include the tumor in the differential diagnosis and help avoid misdiagnosis. Recognition needs a high index of suspicion, although thoracic FDC sarcoma has a high number of pathological features. The detection of FDC sarcomas should be aided by a greater understanding of their morphologic spectrum and the proper immunostains (D2-40 and clusterin) for differentiation as it is extremely similar to various cancers with histiocytic or dendritic origin. Given this neoplasm's substantial potential for recurrence and metastatic spread, accurate characterization is essential. For management aspect, at present, there are no clear indications or guidelines for surgical treatment alone, adjuvant chemotherapy, or radiotherapy in the case of thoracic FDCS. It is challenging for any institute to amass sufficient knowledge on the proper therapy of these patients because of the low prevalence of this condition. Future efforts at their identification, a more thorough characterization of their clinical behavior; potential causal linkages should benefit from a greater understanding of their morphologic spectrum and the appropriate application of FDC markers for any unusual-appearing tumors.

Acknowledgements

Dr. Maria Paul (Senior Resident, Department of Anaesthesiology and Critical Care, Vardhman Mahavir Medical College and Safdarjung Hospital, New Delhi) sketched the image showing how follicular dendritic cells function (**Figure 1**), and I would like to extend my deepest gratitude to her.

Conflict of interest

None of the authors have any conflict of interest.

Abbreviation

FDC	follicular dendritic cell
FDCS	follicular dendritic cell sarcoma
LCH	langerhans cell histiocytosis

PMN	primary malignant neoplasm
EBV	Epstein-Barr virus
HHV-8	human herpesvirus 8
CXCL13	C-X-C motif chemokine ligand 13
BAFF	B activating factor
TLR4	toll-like receptor 4
NF-kB	nuclear factor kappa beta
MAPK	mitogen-activated protein kinase
EGFR	epidermal growth factor receptor
IPT	inflammatory pseudotumor
HV-CD	hyaline-vascular subtype of Castleman disease
IDCS	Interdigitating Dendritic Cell Sarcomas
GIST	gastrointestinal stromal tumor
IMT	inflammatory myofibroblastic tumor
ALK1	anaplastic lymphoma kinase-1
FDCSP	FDC secreted protein
SRGN	serglycin
VAC	vincristine, doxorubicin, and cyclophosphamide
ICE/IE	ifosfamide and etoposide+/−carboplatin
VEGF	vascular endothelial growth factor
OS	overall survival

Author details

Vinay V.* and Priya Sharma
Department of Pulmonary, Critical Care and Sleep Medicine, All India Institute of Medical Sciences (AIIMS), Patna, Bihar, India

*Address all correspondence to: docvinayv@gmail.com

References

[1] Swerdlow SH, Campo E, Pileri SA, Lee Harris N, Stein H, Siebert R, et al. The 2016 revision of the World Health Organization classification of lymphoid neoplasms. Blood. 2016;**127**(20):2375-2390

[2] Emile JF, Abla O, Fraitag S, Horne A, Haroche J, Donadieu J, et al. Revised classification of histiocytoses and neoplasms of the macrophage-dendritic cell lineages. Blood. 2016;**127**(22):2672

[3] Monda L, Warnke R, Rosai J. A primary lymph node malignancy with features suggestive of dendritic reticulum cell differentiation. A report of 4 cases. The American Journal of Pathology. 1986;**122**(3):562

[4] Perez-Ordonez B, Rosai J. Follicular dendritic cell tumor: Review of the entity. Seminars in Diagnostic Pathology. 1998;**15**

[5] Pileri SA, Grogan TM, Harris NL, Banks P, Campo E, Chan JKC, et al. Tumours of histiocytes and accessory dendritic cells: An immunohistochemical approach to classification from the International Lymphoma Study Group based on 61 cases. Histopathology. 2002;**41**

[6] Saygin C, Uzunaslan D, Ozguroglu M, Senocak M, Tuzuner N. Dendritic cell sarcoma: A pooled analysis including 462 cases with presentation of our case series. Critical Reviews in Oncology/Hematology. 2013;**88**(2):253-271

[7] Chan JKC. Proliferative lesions of follicular dendritic (Cells: An overview, including a detailed account of follicular dendritic cell sarcoma): A neoplasm with many faces and uncommon etiologic associations. Advances in Anatomic Pathology. 1997;**4**(6)

[8] Duan GJ, Wu YL, Sun H, Lang L, Chen ZW, Yan XC. Primary follicular dendritic cell sarcoma of the urinary bladder: The first case report and potential diagnostic pitfalls. Diagnostic Pathology. 2017;**12**(1)

[9] Perkins SM, Shinohara ET. Interdigitating and follicular dendritic cell sarcomas: A SEER analysis. American Journal of Clinical Oncology: Cancer Clinical Trials. 2013;**36**

[10] Fassina A, Marino F, Poletti A, Rea F, Pennelli N, Ninfo V. Follicular dendritic cell tumor of the mediastinum. Annals of Diagnostic Pathology. 2001;**5**(6):361-367

[11] Shah RN, Ozden O, Yeldandi A, Peterson L, Rao S, Laskin WB. Follicular dendritic cell tumor presenting in the lung: A case report. Human Pathology. 2001;**32**(7):745-749

[12] Leipsic JA, McAdams HP, Sporn TA. Follicular dendritic cell sarcoma of the mediastinum. American Journal of Roentgenology-New Series. 2007;**188**(6):1694

[13] Denning KL, Olson PR, Maley Richard HJ, Flati VR, Myers JL, SilvermanJF.Primarypulmonaryfollicular dendritic cell neoplasm: A case report and review of the literature. Archives of Pathology & Laboratory Medicine. 2009;**133**(4):643-647

[14] Bushan K. Follicular dendritic cell sarcoma mediastinum-a case report. Indian Journal of Surgical Oncology. 2014;**5**(4):290-292

[15] Lee BE, Korst RJ, Taskin M. Right pneumonectomy for resection of a posterior mediastinal follicular dendritic cell sarcoma arising from Castleman's

disease. The Annals of Thoracic Surgery. 2014;**97**(4):e101-e103

[16] Butler J, Yessayan L, Simoff M. Endobronchial follicular dendritic cell sarcoma. Chest. 2015;**148**(4):539A

[17] Wang R, Han W, Qi L, Shan L, Wang Z, Wang L. Extranodal follicular dendritic cell sarcoma: A clinicopathological report of four cases and a literature review. Oncology Letters. 2015;**9**(1):391-398

[18] Miyoshi R, Sonobe M, Miyamoto E, Date H. Completely resected follicular dendritic cell sarcoma of the posterior mediastinum: Report of a case. Surgery Case Report. 2016;**2**(1)

[19] Sifuentes FUP, Teran SM, Contreras E, Carrera-Ceron R, Bolanos F. Follicular dendritic cell sarcoma in the posterior mediastinum. Chest. 2018;**154**(4):36A

[20] Xu H, Chen B, Jiang C, Yang Z, Wang K. Follicular dendritic cell sarcoma in the right chest wall: A case report. Medicine. 2020;**99**(35)

[21] Ilonen IK, Meltzer AJ, Ellozy S, Bains MS, Huang J. Follicular dendritic cell sarcoma of the chest. The Annals of Thoracic Surgery. 2022;**113**(4):e263-e266

[22] He H, Xue Q, Tan F, Yang L, Wang X, Gao Y, et al. A rare case of primary pulmonary inflammatory pseudotumor-like follicular dendritic cell sarcoma successfully treated by lobectomy. Annals of Translational Medicine. 2021;**9**(1)

[23] Li SH, Dong B, Wu CL, Li ZH, Qi Y. Primary lung follicular dendritic cell sarcoma with rare paraneoplastic pemphigus: A case report. 2022. DOI: 10.21203/rs.3.rs-1780663/v1. Available from: https://www.researchsquare.com/article/rs-1780663/latest

[24] Vinay V, Bansal S, Purwar P, Dewan RK, Verma P, Mullick S, et al. Thoracic follicular dendritic cell sarcoma – An outlandish presentation of a rare tumour with review of literature. Monaldi Archives for Chest Disease. 2023;**93**(2)

[25] Chan JKC. WHO Classification of Tumors of Haematopoietic and Lymphoid Tissues. Vol. 2. IARC Publications; 2008. p. 285

[26] Muppidi JR, Lu E, Cyster JG. The G protein-coupled receptor P2RY8 and follicular dendritic cells promote germinal center confinement of B cells, whereas S1PR3 can contribute to their dissemination. The Journal of Experimental Medicine. 2015;**212**(13):2213-2222

[27] Krautler NJ, Kana V, Kranich J, Tian Y, Perera D, Lemm D, et al. Follicular dendritic cells emerge from ubiquitous perivascular precursors. Cell. 2012;**150**(1)

[28] Maximow A. Bindegewebe und blutbildende Gewebe. Springer; 1927. pp. 232-583. Available from: https://link.springer.com/chapter/10.1007/978-3-642-66441-0_2

[29] Mitchell J, Abbot A. Ultrastructure of the antigen-retaining reticulum of lymph node follicles as shown by high-resolution autoradiography. Nature. 1965;**208**

[30] Foucar K, Foucar E. The mononuclear phagocyte and immunoregulatory effector (M-PIRE) system: Evolving concepts. Seminars in Diagnostic Pathology. 1990;**7**

[31] Tew JG, Kosco MH, Burton GF, Szakal AK. Follicular dendritic cells as accessory cells. Immunological Reviews. 1990;**117**(1):185-211

[32] Kosco MH, Gray D. Signals involved in germinal center

reactions. Immunological Reviews. 1992;**126**(1):63-76

[33] Wang X, Rodda LB, Bannard O, Cyster JG. Integrin-mediated interactions between B cells and follicular dendritic cells influence germinal center B cell fitness. The Journal of Immunology. 2014;**192**(10)

[34] Heesters BA, Myers RC, Carroll MC. Follicular dendritic cells: Dynamic antigen libraries. Nature Reviews. Immunology. 2014;**14**

[35] Bharadwaj H, Freeman J. EBV+ inflammatory pseudotumor-like follicular/fibroblastic dendritic cell sarcoma: An uncommon and challenging tumor. American Journal of Clinical Pathology. 2020;**154**(Supplement_1)

[36] Lee IJ, Kim SC, Kim HS, Bang D, Yang WI, Jung WH, et al. Paraneoplastic pemphigus associated with follicular dendritic cell sarcoma arising from Castleman's tumor. Journal of the American Academy of Dermatology. 1999;**40** (2 II Suppl.)

[37] Facchetti F, Lorenzi L. Follicular dendritic cells and related sarcoma. Seminars in Diagnostic Pathology. 2016;**33**(5):262-276

[38] Facchetti F, Simbeni M, Lorenzi L. Follicular dendritic cell sarcoma. Pathologica. 2021;**113**(5):316-329

[39] Andersen EF, Paxton CN, O'Malley DP, Louissaint A, Hornick JL, Griffin GK, et al. Genomic analysis of follicular dendritic cell sarcoma by molecular inversion probe array reveals tumor suppressor-driven biology. Modern Pathology. 2017;**30**(9):1321-1334

[40] Griffin GK, Sholl LM, Lindeman NI, Fletcher CDM, Hornick JL. Targeted genomic sequencing of follicular dendritic cell sarcoma reveals recurrent alterations in NF-κB regulatory genes. Modern Pathology. 2016;**29**(1)

[41] Go H, Jeon YK, Huh J, Choi SJ, Choi YD, Cha HJ, et al. Frequent detection of BRAFV600E mutations in histiocytic and dendritic cell neoplasms. Histopathology. 2014;**65**(2):261-272

[42] Cheuk W, Chan JKC, Shek TWH, Chang JH, Tsou MH, Yuen NWF, et al. Inflammatory pseudotumor-like follicular dendritic cell tumor: A distinctive low-grade malignant intra-abdominal neoplasm with consistent Epstein-Barr virus association. The American Journal of Surgical Pathology. 2001;**25**(6):721-731

[43] Nayler SJ, Taylor L, Cooper K. HHV-8 is not associated with follicular dendritic cell tumours. Journal of Clinical Pathology – Molecular Pathology. 1998;**51**(3)

[44] Starr JS, Attia S, Joseph RW, Menke D, Casler J, Smallridge RC. Follicular dendritic cell sarcoma present ing as a thyroid mass. Journal of Clinical Oncology. 2015;**33**(17)

[45] Tian X, Xu J, Fletcher C, Hornick JL, Dorfman DM. Expression of enhancer of zeste homolog 2 (EZH2) protein in histiocytic and dendritic cell neoplasms with evidence for p-ERK1/2-related, but not MYC-or p-STAT3-related cell signaling. Modern Pathology. 2018;**31**(4)

[46] Vermi W, Giurisato E, Lonardi S, Balzarini P, Rossi E, Medicina D, et al. Ligand-dependent activation of EGFR in follicular dendritic cells sarcoma is sustained by local production of cognate ligands. Clinical Cancer Research. 2013;**19**(18):5027-5038

[47] Li XQ, Cheuk W, Lam PWY, Wang Z, Loong F, Yeong ML, et al.

Inflammatory pseudotumor-like follicular dendritic cell tumor of liver and spleen: Granulomatous and eosinophil-rich variants mimicking inflammatory or infective lesions. The American Journal of Surgical Pathology. 2014;**38**(5):646-653

[48] Gong S, Auer I, Duggal R, Pittaluga S, Raffeld M, Jaffe ES. Epstein-Barr virus–associated inflammatory pseudotumor presenting as a colonic mass. Human Pathology. 2015;**46**(12):1956-1961

[49] Choe JY, Go H, Jeon YK, Yun JY, Kim YA, Kim HJ, et al. Inflammatory pseudotumor-like follicular dendritic cell sarcoma of the spleen: A report of six cases with increased IgG4-positive plasma cells. Pathology International. 2013;**63**(5):245-251

[50] Pan ST, Cheng CY, Lee NS, Liang PI, Chuang SS. Follicular dendritic cell sarcoma of the inflammatory pseudotumor-like variant presenting as a colonic polyp. Korean Journal of Pathology. 2014;**48**(2):140-145

[51] Chen Y, Shi H, Li H, Zhen T, Han A. Clinicopathological features of inflammatory pseudotumour-like follicular dendritic cell tumour of the abdomen. Histopathology. 2016;**68**(6):858-865

[52] Liu KL, Shen JL, Yang CS, Chen YJ. Paraneoplastic pemphigus as the first manifestation of follicular dendritic cell sarcoma. Journal der Deutschen Dermatologischen Gesellschaft. 2014;**12**(1):68-71

[53] Lu T, Song B, Pu H, Li X, Chen Q, Yang C. Paraneoplastic pemphigus and myasthenia gravis as the first manifestations of a rare case of pancreatic follicular dendritic cell sarcoma: CT findings and review of literature. BMC Gastroenterology. 2019;**19**(1)

[54] Chow SCY, Yeung ECL, Ng CSH, Wong RHL, Fai To K, Wan IYP. Mediastinal follicular dendritic cell sarcoma with paraneoplastic pemphigus. Asian Cardiovascular & Thoracic Annals. 2015;**23**(6):732-734

[55] Garza-Chapa JI, Ocampo- Garza J, Vázquez-Herrera NE, Miranda-MaldonadoIC,Rendón-RamírezE, González-Chávez JM, et al. Paraneoplastic pemphigus associated with primary pulmonar follicular dendritic cell sarcoma showing good response to treatment. Journal of the European Academy of Dermatology and Venereology. 2016;**30**(3):465-467

[56] Zhuang JY, Zhang FF, Li QW, Chen YF. Intra-abdominal inflammatory pseudotumor-like follicular dendritic cell sarcoma associated with paraneoplastic pemphigus: A case report and review of the literature. World Journal of Clinical Cases. 2020;**8**(14):3097-3107

[57] Lin O, Frizzera G. Angiomyoid and follicular dendritic cell proliferative lesions in Castleman's disease of hyaline-vascular type: A study of 10 cases. The American Journal of Surgical Pathology. 1997;**21**(11):1295-1306

[58] Phrathep DD, Healey KD, Anthony S, Fives KR, Boshkos MC, Galani R. Mediastinal follicular dendritic cell sarcoma with underlying Sjogren's syndrome. Cureus. 2023;**4**:1

[59] Shia J, Chen W, Tang LH, Carlson DL, Qin J, Guillem JG, et al. Extranodal follicular dendritic cell sarcoma: Clinical, pathologic, and histogenetic characteristics of an underrecognized disease entity. Virchows Archiv. 2006;**449**(2):148-158

[60] Duan GJ, Wu F, Zhu J, Guo DY, Zhang R, Shen LL, et al. Extranodal follicular dendritic cell sarcoma of the pharyngeal region: A potential diagnostic pitfall, with literature review. American Journal of Clinical Pathology. 2010;**133**(1):49-58

[61] Pathology Outlines. Follicular dendritic cell sarcoma (FDCS). Available from: https://www.pathologyoutlines.com/topic/lymphnodesfdcsarcoma.html [Accessed: Aug 18, 2023]

[62] Wu A, Pullarkat S. Follicular dendritic cell sarcoma. Archives of Pathology & Laboratory Medicine. 2016;**140**(2):186-190

[63] Li Y, Yang X, Tao L, Zeng W, Zuo M, Li S, et al. Challenges in the diagnosis of Epstein-Barr virus-positive inflammatory follicular dendritic cell sarcoma: Extremely wide morphologic spectrum and immunophenotype. The American Journal of Surgical Pathology. 2023;**47**(4):476-489

[64] Lorenzi L, Döring C, Rausch T, Benes V, Lonardi S, Bugatti M, et al. Identification of novel follicular dendritic cell sarcoma markers, FDCSP and SRGN, by whole transcriptome sequencing. Oncotarget. 2017;**8**(10):16463

[65] Massoth LR, Hung YP, Ferry JA, Hasserjian RP, Nardi V, Nielsen GP, et al. Histiocytic and dendritic cell sarcomas of hematopoietic origin share targetable genomic alterations distinct from follicular dendritic cell sarcoma. The Oncologist. 2021;**26**(7):e1263-e1272

[66] Gounder M, Desai V, Kuk D, Agaram N, Arcila M, Durham B, et al. Impact of surgery, radiation and systemic therapy on the outcomes of patients with dendritic cell and histiocytic sarcomas. European Journal of Cancer. 2015;**51**(16):2413-2422

[67] Jain P, Milgrom SA, Patel KP, Nastoupil L, Fayad L, Wang M, et al. Characteristics, management, and outcomes of patients with follicular dendritic cell sarcoma. British Journal of Haematology. 2017;**178**(3):403-412

[68] Conry RM. Response of follicular dendritic cell sarcoma to gemcitabine and docetaxel: Report of two cases and literature review. Clin Sarcoma Res. 2014;**4**(1)

[69] Alfaro C, Suarez N, Gonzalez A, Solano S, Erro L, Dubrot J, et al. Influence of bevacizumab, sunitinib and sorafenib as single agents or in combination on the inhibitory effects of VEGF on human dendritic cell differentiation from monocytes. British Journal of Cancer. 2009;**100**(7):1111-1119

[70] Chen T, Gopal P. Follicular dendritic cell sarcoma. Archives of Pathology & Laboratory Medicine. 2017;**141**(4):596-599

Chapter 4

Emerging Mesenchymal Tumors

Yves-Marie Robin

Abstract

Two new soft tissue entities are described. First, GL1-altered epitheloid mesenchymal tumors comprise two reported molecular subtypes: one with GLI1 fusion and the other with GLI1 amplification, both of which show increased expression of GLI1 RNAm. While most tumors described are malignant, a small subset provisionally termed distinctive nested glomoid neoplasm pursue an indolent course even with regional lymph nodes metastatic spread. There is no known association between prognostication and molecular subtype. Second, the so-called pseudoendocrine sarcoma is considered to be a sarcoma of intermediary grade with a morphology reminiscent of neuroendocrine tumors and characterized by recurrent mutations of the B-catenin gene. This lesion occurs more and less in elderly patients and is most often found in paravertebral area, which makes complete resection surgically relatively challenging.

Keywords: sarcoma, soft tissue, GLI1, fusion, amplification, FISH, RNAseq, pseudoendocrine, B-catenin

1. Introduction

Many soft tissue tumors are currently emerging as new diagnostic entities, a substantial number of them being referenced solely according to their characteristic recurrent molecular alterations, such as PRD10-, N1RD-, or KMT2A-rearrangements, to name just a few [1–3], if only because of the considerable morphological overlap that is observed with already classified lesions in the WHO [4] repertoire widening considerably the range of differential diagnoses. The result is also the confirmation of the importance that molecular genetics is gaining with increasing momentum within the diagnostic armamentarium.

This chapter covers two newcomers, GLI1-altered mesenchymal tumors and pseudoendocrine sarcomas, both presenting cytoarchitecturally as small round and epithelioid cell proliferation.

2. GLI1-altered mesenchymal neoplasms

2.1 General considerations

GLI1 (or Glioma-associated oncogene homolog 1) is a zinc finger-type transcription factor of the krüpell family of proteins playing a distinctive role as a downstream effector in the terminal region of the hedgehog pathway. Among the three known

IntechOpen

isoforms of GLI (GLI1, 2, and 3), GLI1 appears to single out as the only one entirely engaged in transcriptional activation behavior [5, 6]. Alterations of the gene lead to the recognition of two molecular subtypes of the generally small round epithelioid cell tumor with uniform morphology currently encountered and forwarded as emerging lesions, those with amplification and those with fusions. Among the cases thus far reported, our assessment shows that roughly two-thirds belong to the fusion subtype and one-third to the amplified subtype.

The first description of a GLI1-altered mesenchymal tumor dates from 2004 harboring the translocation t(7; 12) with fusion of GLI1 with the ubiquitous B-actin gene (GLI1::ACTB) [7]. This was a lesion of spindle cell morphology labeled as pericytoma or of pericytic phenotype described in soft tissue, bone, and stomach. Although appearing "myopericytomatous" with perivascular features, it is nevertheless distinct from classic myopericytoma at least at the molecular level where the latter exhibits a quite different gene profile characteristic of its pathogenetic make-up: recurrent mutations of PDGFRB that define myopericytomatosis and myofibroma as well [4]. Subsequently, two non-myopericytomatous lesions with GLI1 fusions were classified, located in the gastric wall: one benign with spindle cell morphology, plexiform fibromyxoma [8, 9] and the other malignant and biphasic, gastroblastoma [10].

2.2 Clinical aspects (including prognostication) and gross pathology

Characterization of emerging GLI1-altered tumors is ongoing and combines multifactorial features [11–22]. Their occurrence spans the broadest possible age group between 1 and 80 years, the mean age being 35–41 years, with roughly equal frequency in males and females.

Primary tumors can involve practically any site including soft tissue (trunk including chest wall and abdomino-pelvic regions, limbs, and extremities), head, and neck representing globally 40% of cases (of which around 75% target specifically the tongue), the viscera (lung, endometrium, ovary, kidney, genito-urinary region, and gastro-instestinal tract) and bone such as the tibia, vertebrae, or the scapula.

Based on the published data, we find that 82% of cases are reportedly malignant, with diverse metastatic sites, the most frequently involved being the brain, lung, and lymph nodes. Whereas the remaining 18%, conveniently and provisionally coined "Distinctive Glomoid Nested Tumors," have been observed to pursue an indolent course with no metastasis and no tumor-induced death. If local recurrences have been documented, they are presumably due to too narrowly obtained safe margins at excision. No difference in prognosis related to a particular molecular alteration has been noted thus far.

Tumors may be deep-seated or superficial arising in the subcutis. They may measure anywhere from 0.9 to 12 cm, the median size being 3–5 cm. They are generally lobulated, compact or partially cystic, white-colored, or sometimes hemorrhagic. Overtly malignant cases have infiltrative borders.

2.3 Light microscopy features

Tumors are generally composed of multinodular sheets of nested or trabecular small round monotonous cells (**Figure 1**) with more or less vesicular nuclei or lightly spread chromatin, and separated by fibrous septa. There is possible focal spindling, and only rarely a biphasic architecture. On most occasions, these cells are embedded in a delicately vascularized stroma, which can be myxoid, conveying a perivascular

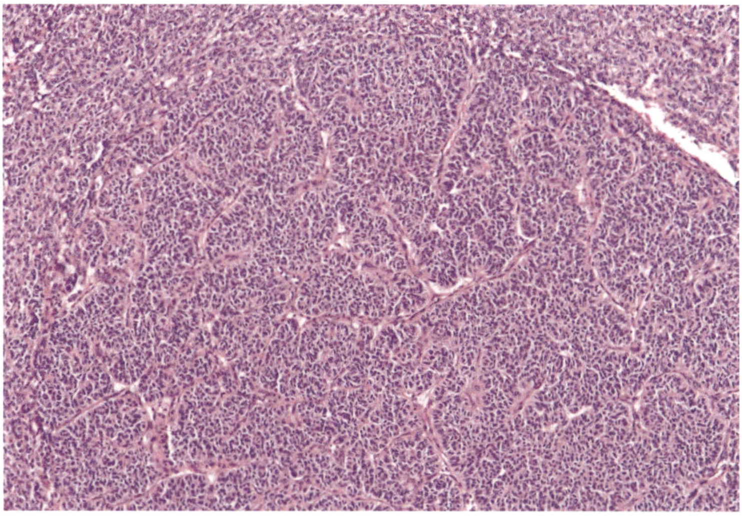

Figure 1.
GLI1-altered mesenchymal tumor- distinctive nested Glomoid neoplasm (courtesy of Dr. D Papke, Brigham and Women's hospital, Harvard Medical School, Boston, USA).

configuration. Necrosis is an eventuality. A very frequent feature is lymphovascular invasion [11, 12, 16, 20, 21].

2.4 Immunohistochemical aspects

No consistent immunophenotypic profile has been described, except the almost constant GLI1 expression (**Figure 2**). Parrack et al. found GLI1 nuclear or nucleo-cytoplasmic tumor positivity with 98% specificity and 91.3% sensitivity using the C1 clone antibody of Santa Cruz in test cohort and control cohort cases [21].

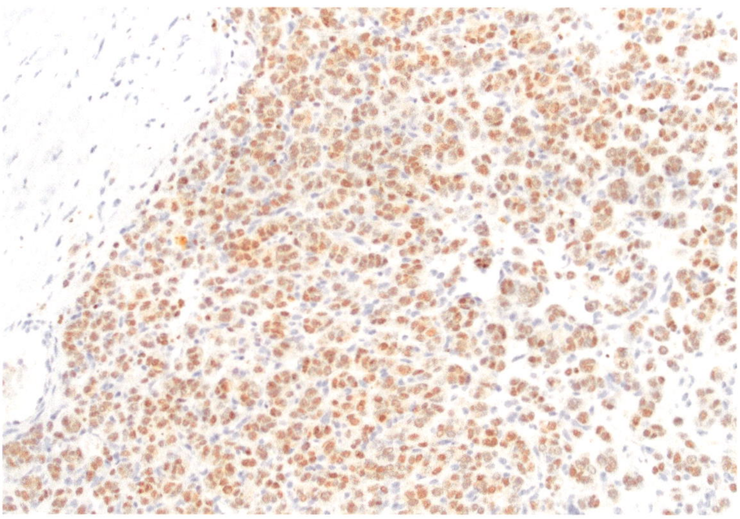

Figure 2.
Diffuse immunohistochemical expression of GLI1 antibody in GLI1-altered mesenchymal tumor (courtesy of Dr. D Papke, Brigham and Women's hospital, Harvard Medical School).

S100 protein and smooth muscle actin immunostaining are observed in a little less than half of cases and keratin AE1-AE3 in 15% of cases, at least focally [11, 13, 20]. Neuroendocrine markers such as CD56 [11, 12] and synaptophysin [14] are reported positive albeit with no clear rationale. More importantly, MdM2 and CDK4 [12, 20] as well as STAT6 [20] have been proven to be not surprisingly overexpressed in GLI1-amplified lesions, the genes coding for these proteins being part of the amplicon 12q13–15 with possible co-amplifications with GLI1.

In tumors arising, especially in the oropharynx and tonsils, P16 is usually positive, probably due to the negative feedback loop whereby Rb silencing by hyperphosphorylation-inducing GLI1-activated cyclin/cyclin dependant kinase complexes leads to P16 overexpression [17]. Thus purportedly GLI1-activated Cyclin D1 can be found to be positive. A number of tumors are immunostain with CD10 and BCOR as well [18].

2.5 Molecular genetics

In GLI1-rearranged tumors, various fusion partners of the gene have been identified by sequencing methods (RNA sequencing), including, for example, ACTB1, PTCH1, FOXO4, PAMR1, HNRNPA1, NEAT1, and QTXNIP. Promoter swapping seems to be the generally accepted mechanism resulting in GLI1 oncogenic activation. GLI1 rearrangements as well as amplifications are readily highlighted by fluorescent *in situ* hybridization (FISH) techniques. Some cases presumably show rearrangement and concomitant amplification of the gene with discordant FISH and RNAseq results and attributed by some authors to genetic instability phenomenon [14].

Moreover, since GLI1 shares with DDIT3 the locus 12q13.3, some seven authors propose re-arrangements of DDIT3 as observed with some commercial break-apart probes (VYSIS or CytoCELL) as a surrogate marker for GLI1 rearrangement [17].

GLI1 highly amplified lesions can harbor co-amplifications not only of some neighboring genes but of the whole oncogene-rich amplicon 12q13–15 as demonstrated by molecular karyotyping, the most frequently involved genes being MdM2, CDK4, HMGA2, STAT6, and DDIT3 and much less frequently the genes LRP1, TSPAN31, FRS2, and ARHGEF25 [14].

2.6 Major differential diagnoses

Undifferentiated carcinoma and small round cell sarcomas of unknown differentiation (SRCSUD) represent the bulk of differential diagnoses, including the currently emerging pseudoendocrine sarcoma (cf. infra). In this context, variants of dedifferentiated liposarcoma morphologically similar to SRCSUD must be recognized for they can immunostain for GLI1 [21].

Neuroendocrine tumors (carcinoma, paraganglioma) are to be considered because, like these, GLI1-altered tumors can express CD56 and/or synaptophysin (cf supra par.2.5). Other pitfalls are ossifying fibro-myxoid tumor (nonossifiying variant) neuroblastoma, neuroectodermal tumors, (including melanocytic tumors), PEComa, and glomus tumors. GLI1-altered tumors share with myoepithelioma possible S100 protein positivity. A fairly recent case report describes a myoepithelioma with GLI1 fusion (TUBA1::GLI1) without any other alterations known in classic myoepithelioma [23]. According to our view, if this is confirmed by other reports, it raises at least the possibility of the existence of a lesional continuum between conventional myoepithelioma at one end and GLI1-fusion tumor at the other. High-grade endometrial stromal sarcoma can be a mimic of gynecologically located GLI1-altered tumors inasmuch as both lesions can express Cyclin D1, CD10, and BCOR (cf supra par.2.5). SDH-deficient gastrointestinal stromal tumor should also be mentioned as a differential diagnosis if consistent with primary tumor location. In head and neck localizations, GLI1- tumor remains an alternative possibility to HPV-induced oropharyngeal neuroendocrine carcinoma sharing with it P16 positivity, and to sialoblastoma notably in the pediatric population.

3. Pseudoendocrine sarcoma

3.1 Clinical aspects (including prognostication) and gross pathology

The mean age of occurrence is 52, with extremes being 29 and 74, thus more in the elderly age group than GLI1-altered tumors [24, 25]. There is a slight predilection for men.

The prevalent localization is the paravertebral region, other areas of the trunk being less frequent (chest wall, buttock, and groin) as well as head and neck sites.

This sarcoma of unknown differentiation is currently considered to be a tumor of intermediate malignancy with 43% risk of local recurrence and 21% risk of metastatic spread, knowing that these may be eventually underestimated. Frequent metastatic sites are lung and lymph nodes.

Tumors are deep-seated and their size varies from 2 to 19 cm, the median size being around 6 cm. They are grossly described as compact and hemorrhagic growths.

3.2 Light microscopy and ultrastructural features

The term "pseudoendocrine" refers to the histological architecture reminiscent of well-differentiated neuroendocrine carcinoma [24–26]. It is generally lobulated, nested, or trabecular like GLI1-altered tumor, packed with small round cells displaying stippled chromatin embedded in a delicately woven stroma (**Figure 3**). Mitoses can be found in great numbers (more than 5 per high power field). No necrosis has been thus far recorded. Electron microscopy undertaken in two tumors shows no

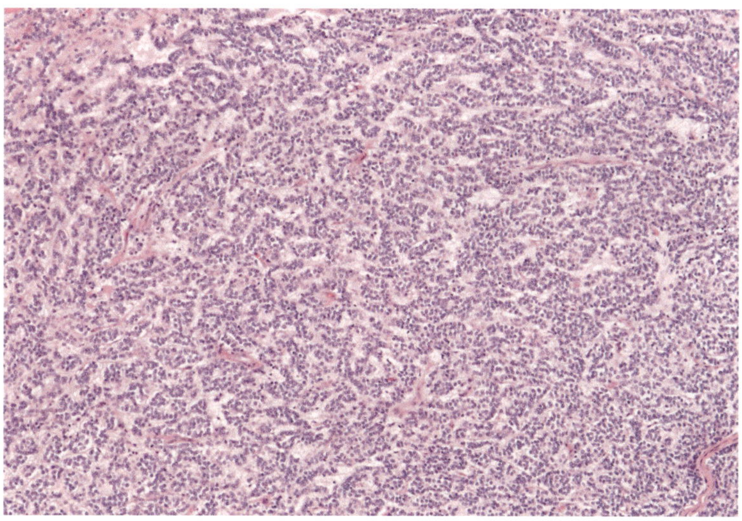

Figure 3.
Pseudoendocrine sarcoma: Endocrine-like morphology in light microscopy (courtesy of Dr. D Papke, Brighamn and Women's hospital, Harvard Medical School, Boston USA).

characteristic neurosecretory granules in favor of neuroendocrine differentiation, but intercellular junctions with cytoplasmic cell processes [27]. Other occasional features include pseudoglandular aspects, calcifications, and stromal hyaline globules. Tumors have generally poorly circumscribed margins.

3.3 Immunohistochemical aspects

Tumors show diffuse nuclear B-catenin positivity in 95% of cases (**Figure 4**) and S100 protein reactivity (**Figure 5**), at least focal, in 40% of cases. Desmin is reported

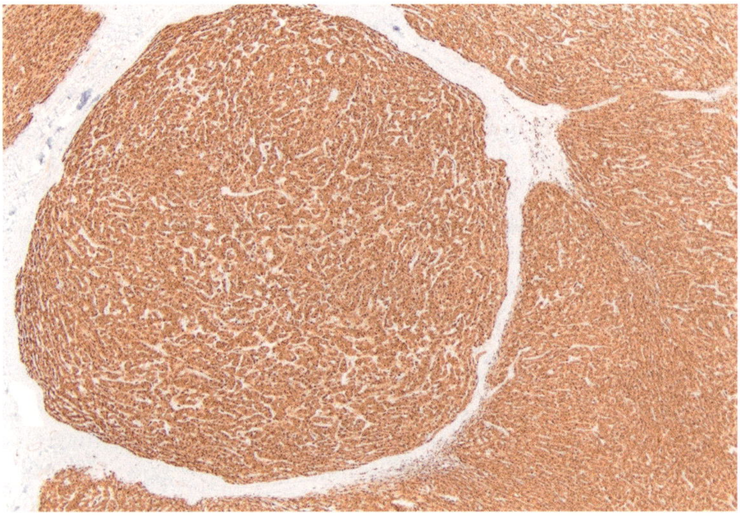

Figure 4.
Diffuse B-catenin immunohistochemical expression in pseudoendocrine sarcoma (courtesy of Dr. D Papke, Brighman and Women's hospital, Harvard Medical School, Boston, USA).

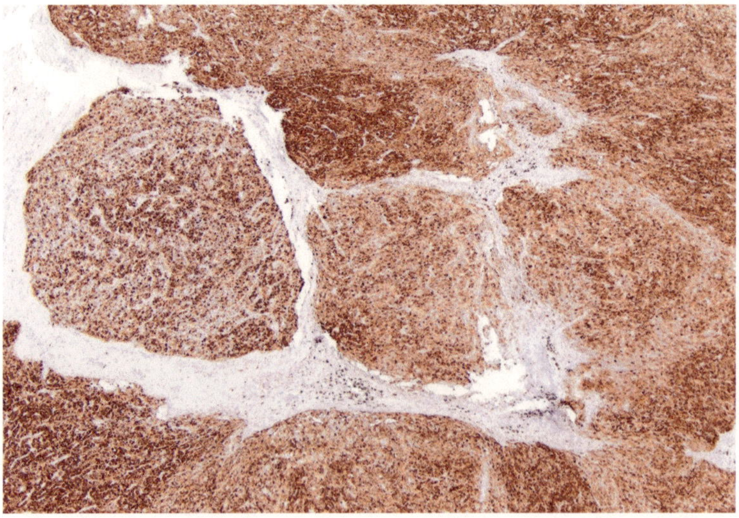

Figure 5.
Diffuse S-100 protein immunohistochemical expression in pseudoendocrine sarcoma (courtesy of Dr. D Papke, Brighman and Women's hospital, Harvard Medical School, Boston, USA).

positive in slightly less than 30% of cases and CD34 in 25% of tumors. Expression of keratin and/or neuroendocrine markers is not characteristic features [24–26].

3.4 Molecular genetics

Recurrent B-catenin gene mutations identified by DNA sequencing methods are the hallmark of this tumor such as D32H, S33C, S331f, S37C, and S37F [24]. Their range does not generally overlap with that of desmoid fibromatosis but exceptionally the latter may harbor the D32H mutation. No other recurrent abnormality is found with RNA seq and no wild-type variant has been thus far discussed in the literature.

3.5 Differential diagnoses

The differential diagnoses are virtually the same as for GLI1-altered tumors (cf. supra par.2.6). It should nonetheless be emphasized that neither speckled chromatin nor B-catenin mutation is a known feature of any other known round cell sarcoma.

We add in this category of differential diagnoses pancreatic and ovarian solid pseudo-papillary tumors, which are small round cell non-sarcomatous tumors with characteristic b-catenin nuclear expression as well [28].

4. Conclusion

GLI1-altered mesenchymal round epithelioid cell tumors are ubiquitous and can be malignant generally speaking or more rarely of limited malignant potential irrespective of the oncogenic molecular abnormality involved, fusion, or amplification. Fusion tumors are more frequent than amplified ones. Immunohistochemistry with anti-GLI1 antibody is the simplest method of choice to distinguish these tumors from their potential mimics.

Pseudoendocrine sarcoma is a descriptive term with no common grounds with endocrine differentiation, considered to be a rare sarcoma of intermediate grade most frequently located in the paravertebral region. Its hallmark is a recurrent B-catenin mutation and immunohistochemical nuclear expression. Literature is still scarce with only around 24 cases reported.

Author details

Yves-Marie Robin
Centre Oscar Lambret Cancer Center, Biopatholoy Wing, Lille, France

*Address all correspondence to: ym-robin@o-lambret.fr

References

[1] Puls F, Pillay N, Fagman H, et al. PRDM10-rearranged soft tissue tumor: A clinicopathologic study of 9 cases. The American Journal of Surgical Pathology. 2019;**43**(4):504-513. DOI: 10.1097/PAS.0000000000001207

[2] Lacambra MD, Antonescu CR, Chow C, et al. Expanding the spectrum of mesenchymal neoplasms with NR1D1-rearrangement. Genes, Chromosomes & Cancer. 2022;**61**(7):420-426. DOI: 10.1002/gcc.23032

[3] Folpe A. 'I can't keep up !': An update on advances in soft itssue pathology occurring after the publicaion of the 2020 world health organization classification of soft tissue and bone tumors. Histopathology. 2022;**80**:54-75. DOI: 10.1111/his.14460

[4] Soft tissue and bone tumors. In: WHO Classification of Tumors. Editorial Board, Ed. 5th ed. Lyon: IARC Press; 2020

[5] Mendelsohn J, Howley PM, Israel MA et al. The Molecular Basis of Cancer. 3rd ed. Philadelphia, PA: Saunders; 2008

[6] Habib JG, O'Shaughnessy JA. The hedgehog pathway in triple-negative breast cancer. Cancer Medicine. 2016;**5**(10):2989-3006

[7] Dahlen A, Fletcher CD, Mertens F, et al. Activation of the GLI oncogene (Gliome-associated oncogene 1) through fusion with the beta-actin gene (ACTB) in a group of distinctive pericytic neoplasms: Pericytoma with t(7; 12). The American Journal of Pathology. 2004;**164**:1645-1653

[8] Miettinen M, Makhlouf HR, Sobin LH, et al. Plexiform fibromyxoma, a distinctive benign gastric antral neoplasm not to be confused with a myxoid GIST. The American Journal of Surgical Pathology. 2009;**33**:1624-1632

[9] Spans L, Fletcher CD, Antonescu et al. Recurrent MALAT-GLI1 oncogenic fusion and GLI1 up-regulation define a subset of plexiform fibromyxoma. The Journal of Pathology 2016; 239:335-343. DOI: 10.1002/path.4730

[10] Graham RP, Nair AA, Davila JL, et al. Gastroblastoma harbors a recurrent somatic MALAT1-GLI1 fusion gene. Modern Pathology. 2017;**30**:1443-1452. DOI: 10.1038/modpathol.2017.68

[11] Antonescu CR, Agaram NP, Sung YS, et al. A distinct malignant epithelioid neoplasm with GLI1 gene rearrangements, frequent S100 protein expression, and metastatic potential: Expanding the spectrum of pathologic entities with ACTB/MALAT1/PTCH1-GLI1 fusions. The American Journal of Surgical Pathology. 2018;**42**(4):1. DOI: 10.1097/PAS.0000000000001010

[12] Agaram NP, Zhang L, Sung YS, et al. GLI1-amplifications expands the spectrum of soft tissue neoplasms defined by GLI1 gene fusions. Modern Pathology. 2019;**32**(11):1617-1626. DOI: 10.1038/s41379-019-0293-x

[13] Kerr DA, Pinto A, Subhawong TK, et al. Pericytoma with t(7; 12) and ACTB-GLI fusion: Réévaluation of an unusual entity and its relationship to the spectrum of GLI1 fusion-related neoplasms. The American Journal of Surgical Pathology. 2019;**43**(12):682-1692. DOI: 10.1097/PAS.0000000000001360

[14] Liu J, Mao R, Lao IW, et al. GLI1-altered mesenchymal tumor:

A clinicopathological and molecular analysis of ten additional cases of an emerging entity. Virchows Archiv. 2022;**480**(5):1087-1099. DOI: 10.1007/s00428-021-03224-0

[15] Punjabi LS, Goh CHR, Sittampalam K. Expanding the spectrum of GLI1-altered mesenchymal tumors-a high-grade uterine sarcoma harboring a novel PAMR1: GLI1 fusion and literature reviez of GLI1-altered mesenchymal neoplasms of the gynecologic tract. Genes, Chromosomes & Cancer. 2023;**62**:107-117. DOI: 10.1002/gcc.23099

[16] Papke DJ Jr, Dickson BC, Oliveira AM, et al. Distinctive nested glomoid neoplasm: Clinicopathologic analysis of 20 cases of a mesenchymal neoplasm with frequent GLI1 alterations and indolent behavior. al. The American Journal of Surgical Pathology. 2023;**47**(1):12-24. DOI: 10.1097/PAS.0000000000001979

[17] Palsgrove DN, Rooper LM, Stevens TM, et al. GLI1-altered soft tissue tumors of the head and neck: Frequent oropharyngeal involvement, p16 Immunoreactivity, and detectable alterations by DDIT3 break apart FISH. Head and Neck Pathology. 2022;**16**(4):1146-1156. Epub Aug 06, 2022. DOI: 10.1007/s12105-022-01476-z

[18] Argani P, Boyraz B, Oliva E, et al. GLI1 gene alterations in neoplasms of the genitourinary and gynecologic tract. The American Journal of Surgical Pathology. 2022;**46**(5):677-687. DOI: 10.1097/PAS.0000000000001844

[19] Jessurun J, Orr C, McNulty S, et al. *GLI1*-rearranged enteric tumor. Expanding the Spectrum of gastrointestinal neoplasms with *GLI1* gene fusions. The American Journal of Surgical Pathology. 2023;**47**(1):65-73. DOI: 10.1097/PAS.0000000000001950

[20] Xu B, Chang K, Folpe A et al Head and neck mesenchymal neoplasms with *GLI1* gene alterations. A pathologic entity with distinct histologic features and potential for distant metastasis. The American Journal of Surgical Pathology 44(6):p 729-737, 2020. DOI: 10.1097/PAS.0000000000001439

[21] Parrack PH, Mariño-Enríquez A, Fletcher CDM, et al. *GLI1* immunohistochemistry distinguishes mesenchymal neoplasms with *GLI1* alterations from morphologic mimics. The American Journal of Surgical Pathology. 2023;**47**(4):453-460. DOI: 10.1097/PAS.0000000000002018

[22] Klubickova N et al. Epithelioid soft tissue neoplasm of the soft palate with a PTCH1-GLI1 fusion: A case report and review of the literature. Head and Neck Pathology. 2022;**16**(5):621-630. DOI: 10.1007/s12105-021-01388-4

[23] Liu YJ, Wagner MJ, Kim EY, et al. TUBA1A-GLI1 fusion in a soft tissue myoepithelial neoplasm. Human Pathology: Case Reports. 2021;**24**:1-5. DOI: 10.1016/j.ehpc.2021.200497

[24] Papke DJ Jr, Dickson BC, Sholl L, Fletcher CDM. Pseudoendocrine sarcoma: Clinicopathologic analysis of 23 cases of a distinctive soft tissue neoplasm with metastatic potential, recurrent CTNNB1 mutations, and a predilection for truncal locations. The American Journal of Surgical Pathology. 2022;**46**:33-43. DOI: 10.1111/his.14460

[25] Bellan E, Zanco F, Baciorri F, et al. Case report: Pseudoendocrine sarcoma, a clinicopathologic report of a newly described soft tissue neoplasm. Virchows Archiv. 2023;**482**:1057-1063. DOI: 10.1007/s00428-022-03476-4

[26] Karini SS, Gonzalez MF. Paravertebral pseudoendocrine sarcoma.

American Journal of Clinical Pathology. 2022;**158**:S30-S161. DOI: 10.1093/acjp/agac126

[27] Moran JMT, Hung YP, Selig MK, et al. Meningioma-like ultrastructural features of pseudoendocrine sarcoma. The American Journal of Surgical Pathology. 2022;**46**(7):1014-1016. DOI: 10.1097/PAS.0000000000001890

[28] He S, Yang X, Zhou P, et al. Case report: Solid pseudopapillary tumor: An invasive case report of primary ovarian origin and review of the literature. International Journal of Clinical and Experimental Pathology. 2015;**8**(7):8645-8649. Available from: www.ijcep.com/; ISSN:1936-2625/IJCEP0009908

Section 2

Uterine Leiomyoma – Diagnosis and Management

Chapter 5

New Insights into Molecular Pathogenesis of Uterine Fibroids: From the Lab to a Clinician-Friendly Review

Demetrio Larraín and Jaime Prado

Abstract

Uterine fibroids (UFs) (also known as leiomyomas or myomas) are the most common form of benign uterine tumors, affecting 70–80% of women over their lifetime. Although uterine fibroids (UFs) are benign, these lesions cause significant morbidity and represent a major public health concern in reproductive age women. It has been hypothesized that leiomyomas arise from clonal proliferation of a single myometrial cell due to an initial genetic insult. However, these early cytogenetic alterations are insufficient for tumor development. In recent years, many advances have been made in the understanding of molecular mechanisms underlying the pathogenesis of uterine fibroids, and aberrations in several complex signaling pathways have shown to be involved in myoma development. In addition, most of these altered signaling cascades converge in a summative way, making the understanding of myoma biology even more complex. In this chapter, we focus on integrating this new knowledge in a simpler way to make it friendly to the general gynecologist.

Keywords: myoma, genetics, growth factors, theory, signaling, epigenetics, ECM

1. Introduction

Uterine fibroids (UFs) (also known as leiomyomas or myomas) are the most common form of benign uterine tumors, affecting 70–80% of women over their lifetime [1]. Although uterine fibroids (UFs) are benign, these lesions cause significant morbidity and represent a major public health concern in reproductive age women [2]. Leiomyomas are monoclonal tumors that arise from uterine smooth muscle (i.e., the myometrium) [3]. Histologically, leiomyomas are composed of disordered smooth muscle cells, vascular smooth muscle cells, fibroblasts, myofibroblasts and are rich in extracellular matrix (ECM) [4–6]. Despite their high prevalence, the exact pathophysiology of uterine myomas is still unknown, although ethnicity-related data seem to indicate that the prevalence is about three times higher in African-American women. However, some other factors, such as early menarche, nulliparity, heredity, obesity, diabetes, hypertension, exposure to diethylstilbestrol (DES), air pollution, and dietary factors like high-fat diet, alcohol, and vitamin D deficiency, may also be involved in its incidence and development [5, 7, 8].

In recent years, many advances have been made, allowing us to understand the molecular mechanisms underlying the pathogenesis of UFs. The role of myometrial stem cells as tumor-initiating cells (TICs), the contribution of an abnormal ECM to tumor biology, the science of solid-state signaling in growth factors (GFs) metabolism and related pathways, the influence of epigenetic factors, steroid hormones and their receptors, the impact of myofibroblastic differentiation on inflammation and repair processes, and myometrial ischemia in tumor environment, have allowed a better understanding of myoma development and its clinical manifestations, such as abnormal uterine bleeding, dysmenorrhea, and infertility. In this chapter, we focus on integrating this new knowledge in a simpler way to make it friendly to the general gynecologist. However, it is important for better understanding of this chapter that many of the described molecular processes converge, link, and overlap.

2. Myometrial stem cells and myoma development

Somatic stem cells (SSCs) are a subset of cells residing in normal adult tissues that, through asymmetric division, retain their ability to self-renew while producing daughter cells that go on to differentiate and play a role in tissue regeneration and repair. Likewise, TICs are a subset of cells within a tumor cell population, which, also through asymmetric division, retain the ability to reconstitute tumors [9]. Several studies have described the presence of putative SSCs in myometrium (myometrial stem cells) and leiomyomas (leiomyoma stem cells). It has been suggested that several myometrial pathologies, such as UFs, can be attributed to the dysregulation of these SSCs, or that they might have derived from differentiated myometrial cells that acquire stem-like features (TICs) [9–12]. It is hypothesized that leiomyomas originate from somatic mutations in myometrial stem cells which transform them to fibroid progenitor cells (leiomyoma stem cells, TICs), resulting in progressive loss of growth regulation [10, 12]. The tumor grows as genetically abnormal clones of cells derived from a single fibroid progenitor cell (in which the original mutation took place). Although fibroids are clonal in origin, considerable heterogeneity exists, and fibroids vary greatly in size, location, and appearance even within the same uterus. Interestingly, multiple myomas within the same uterus are not clonally related; each myoma arises independently [13]. In addition, fibroids from the same woman grow at different rates, with some regressing, despite a uniform hormonal milieu [14]. Moreover, fibroid characteristics, such as size, location, and ultrasonographic blood flow, do not correlate with fibroid growth, uterine bleeding, or any other symptomatology [14, 15], and therefore, further research is needed to identify biological or molecular factors that determine fibroid behavior.

The cellular composition of clonal fibroids is heterogeneous, including smooth muscle cells, vascular smooth muscle cells, fibroblasts, and myofibroblasts [3]. These phenotypically different clones exhibit differential expression of fibroid-associated genes: CRABP2 (encoding cellular retinoic acid-binding protein 2), PGR (encoding progesterone receptor B), and TGFBR2 (encoding TGF-β3 receptor 2) [4, 16]. These different gene profiles help to explain the heterogeneity of fibroid biology and clinical type.

Although the understanding of human myometrial stem cells is still limited, it is theorized that their population remains undifferentiated in its niche and under the right conditions can contribute to either physiologic (pregnancy) or pathologic processes (leiomyoma) [11].

It has been hypothesized that uterine hypoxia, aberrant methylation, or abnormal estrogen signaling could play a critical role in the transformation of a myometrial stem cell into a TIC [17, 18].

Despite a distinguishing feature of UFs being their dependency on the estrogen and progesterone to grow, leiomyoma stem cells comprised 1% of all tumor cells and they have very low sex steroid hormone receptor levels [9].

Ono et al. [19] studied the biological behavior of leiomyoma stem cells under different conditions, with the use of the side population technique. They concluded that even if leiomyoma stem cells are necessary for *in vivo* growth of UFs, their low estrogen and progesterone receptor levels, and their inability to grow and survive in a steroid hormone-only enrichment culture, suggest that other factors than steroid hormones are necessary for leiomyoma stem cell survival. Interestingly, leiomyoma stem cells had tumorigenic capacity under estrogen and progesterone stimulation when inoculated together with differentiated myometrial cells, demonstrating an indirect paracrine effect of steroid hormones on leiomyoma stem cells *via* the mature (differentiated) neighboring cells (normal myometrial or leiomyoma cells) [19]. Furthermore, leiomyoma stem cells were able to differentiate into uterine leiomyoma cells, gain their same potential of proliferation, and express steroid hormone receptors after coculture with mixed myometrial cells [9, 19].

In summary, it has been proposed that a single myometrial stem cell goes through tumorigenic transformation following a cellular insult (genetic hit) and gives rise to daughter leiomyoma stem cell (TIC), which proliferate, undergo self-renewal, and clonally expand in response to steroid hormones *via* paracrine signaling from surrounding differentiated myometrial and leiomyoma cells.

It has been demonstrated that paracrine activation of the wingless-type (Wnt)/β-catenin pathway mediated by estrogen and progesterone has a critical role in enhancing the growth and proliferation of leiomyoma stem cells [19]. The presence of steroid hormones stimulates the secretion of Wnt ligands from mature myometrium or leiomyoma cells. This induces the nuclear translocation of β-catenin in leiomyoma stem cells, leading to the expression of genes with a critical role in UFs growth and development. This pathway can stimulate the expression of transforming growth factor-β3 (TGF-β3), which induces fibronectin (an ECM protein) expression, cell proliferation, and extracellular matrix accumulation [4, 20] (see below). Then, the development of clinical disease is dependent on a paracrine mechanism and a multistep process from transformation to the fibroid progenitor through to growth acceleration. Even though some cell-related events have been identified, the exact cell of origin of uterine leiomyomas remains unknown.

3. The conception of UFs as a fibrotic/inflammatory disease: the role of myofibroblastic transformation

It is well accepted that menstruation, ovulation, and parturition represent physiological injury that triggers an inflammatory reaction of the uterus, then, demanding tissue repair and remodeling. It has been hypothesized that UFs could be the consequence of an improper inflammatory response and fibrosis development mediated by myofibroblasts [6, 17, 21, 22].

A myofibroblast is a cell phenotype that has the characteristics of a fibroblast and smooth muscle cells and is characterized by the expression of α-smooth muscle actin (α-SMA); therefore, it is a nonmuscle contracting cell [23, 24]. Myofibroblasts drive connective tissue remodeling by combining ECM synthesizing features of fibroblasts with the cytoskeletal characteristics of contractile smooth muscle cells and have been observed in several fibrotic diseases, including systemic sclerosis, glomerulosclerosis, idiopathic pulmonary fibrosis, and liver cirrhosis [24, 25]. Chronic inflammation plays a critical role in fibrosis and tumorigenesis. The pathophysiology of UFs is the same as that of other fibrotic conditions, in which an injury triggers normally quiescent cells to dedifferentiate into a myofibroblast-like, more proliferative phenotype [25].

Myofibroblasts are activated by inflammation, tissue injury, mechanical forces, hypoxia, and oxidative stress. Once activated, myofibroblasts proliferate and produce ECM proteins in the process of wound healing. After finishing this role in tissue repair, these specialized cells lose their contractile activity, decrease α-SMA expression, and disappear by apoptosis [6]. On the other hand, their inappropriate function has been shown to cause fibrosis, creating a collagenous and stiff scar, such as how it occurs in keloids [17, 26]. In the uterus, myofibroblastic transformation could occur from smooth muscle cells, connective tissue fibroblasts, vascular smooth muscle cells, or direct myofibroblastic differentiation of SSCs [17, 27]. Furthermore, the presence of myofibroblasts in UFs has been well documented [6]; then, UFs can be considered as a fibrotic disorder, sharing several characteristics with those of keloids [17].

Cellular transformation into a myofibroblastic phenotype is key to the establishment and progression of fibrogenesis [28]. Several studies have documented a pivotal role of inflammation and myofibroblastic transformation in the pathogenesis of UFs, and it is beginning to be accepted that local chronic inflammation generates a microenvironment that fosters the development of UFs [22]. The consideration of UFs as a chronic inflammatory disease is supported by the presence of high expression of inflammatory cytokines in fibroids, including interleukin (IL)-1, IL-6, IL-13, IL-15, tumor necrosis factor (TNF)-α, granulocyte-macrophage colony-stimulating factor (GM-CSF), and erythropoietin [28]. Moreover, Protic et al. [22] showed the presence of many inflammatory cells, such as macrophages, mast cells, and leukocytes, inside UFs and their surrounding tissues when compared to autologous myometrium distant from the tumor.

Moreover, a recent study by Orciani et al. [29] showed a distinct cytokine expression pattern related to chronic inflammation in leiomyoma progenitor cells (leiomyoma stem cells) that could favor a microenvironment suitable for leiomyoma onset and development. In addition, the authors hypothesized that this upregulated cytokine profile could play a role in adverse obstetric outcomes, including infertility, spontaneous miscarriage, and preterm delivery in women with UFs.

Myofibroblastic differentiation can be triggered by multiple cell pathways, environmental cues, physical factors, such an ECM tension, and a variety of inflammatory molecules including cytokines, steroid hormones, and growth factors released locally by adjacent resident cells [6]. Growth factors are usually carried in the ECM. They are stimulated and then released by mechanical stress or proteolytic cleavage. Then, they migrate to bind to membrane receptors [28]. This phenomenon leads to activation of the intracellular complexes that migrate to the nucleus, thus promoting the transcription or repression of target genes that are involved in fibrosis [30].

The central player of myofibroblastic differentiation is transforming growth factor-β (TGF-β). Transforming growth factor-β1 (TGF-β1) activates fibroblasts by starting α-SMA synthesis leading to myofibroblastic differentiation [31].
This molecular marker, which is not present in a fibroblast, is characteristic of the

new myofibroblastic phenotype and stimulates the contractile properties of myofibroblasts [32]. Expression of α-SMA is a highly regulated process and depends on the presence of TGF-β1 and Activin-A [25].

Although most women experience causes of uterine inflammation, such as reproductive events, they all do not have UFs. This observation suggests that the initiation of myoma development does not solely depend on inflammation. There are other factors that may influence the risk of developing UFs under the chronic inflammatory condition.

4. Genetic aberrations and myoma

A genetic predisposition to UFs appears to be present as a family predisposition has been shown [33]. There is about a 2.5-fold increased risk of developing myomas in first-degree relatives of women with these tumors. Moreover, the diagnosis of UFs is almost twice in monozygotic twins compared to dizygotic twins [34]. Cytogenetically, most of the UFs (60%) are chromosomally normal [35]. However, several recurrent genetic aberrations, related to a variety of tumor-promoting functions, such as DNA repair, apoptosis regulation, modulation of epithelial-mesenchymal transition, and formation of fibroid-like tissues, have been identified in uterine fibroids [5]. Different rates of growth can reflect the different chromosomal abnormalities present in individual tumors. Current research has revealed the existence of four subgroups of UFs, depending on somatic mutations or chromosomal alterations [4]:

4.1 Somatic mutation in the mediator complex subunit 12 gene *(MED12)*

Somatic mutation in the mediator complex subunit 12 gene *(MED12)* is the most frequent mutation found in uterine myomas (70%) and it has been identified only in leiomyoma stem cells but not in normal myometrial stem cells [9, 36]. Therefore, it has been hypothesized that at least one genetic hit may transform a myometrial stem cell into a TIC, which then interacts with the surrounding myometrium to give rise to a UF [5]. However, the role of these mutations is not fully understood. Distinct *MED12* somatic mutations have been detected in different fibroid lesions in the same uterus, but not in all [10, 13]. *MED12* gene encodes one of the components of the mediator complex, which is a group of 26 proteins that work together to regulate gene activity. Mediator complex acts as a transcriptional regulator that bridges DNA regulatory sequences to the RNA polymerase II initiation complex. *MED12* protein is part of several chemical signaling pathways involving cell growth, migration, and differentiation. Aberrant function of *MED12* contributes to tumorigenesis, and it is believed that *MED12* mutation is a driver for stimulating the development of uterine fibroids and genomic instability [10]. In addition, MED12 deficiency inhibits TGF-β signaling by reducing activation of Wnt/β-catenin pathway [37–40]. MED12 mutations have been suggested as a causal agent of UFs [36]; however, direct supportive cause and effect evidence remain lacking.

4.2 Chromosomal rearrangements in high mobility group AT-hook 2 *(HMGA2)* gene

Chromosomal rearrangements in high mobility group AT-hook 2 *(HMGA2)* gene have been identified in 7.5–10% of UFs, and these are the second most common genetic alterations in these tumors [41]. *HMGA* protein functions as an architectural factor and contains structural DNA-binding domains and may act as a transcription-regulating factor. With few exceptions, HMGA2 is expressed in human only during early development and is reduced to undetectable levels of transcription in adult tissues. The expression of *HMGA2* in adult tissues is associated with modulation of epithelial-mesenchymal transition, mesenchymal differentiation, tumor formation, and certain characteristic cancer-promoting mutations, such as inactivation of p53-induced apoptosis. Overexpression of *HMGA2* in myometrial cells may lead to abnormal growth of the myometrial stem cell niche, resulting in fibroid-like tissues [10]. It has been postulated that *MED12* and *HMGA2* mutations were mutually exclusive in fibroids [42], suggesting distinct tumorigenic pathways. However, a recent study reported simultaneous alterations in both genes in 50% of the tumors. The authors concluded that *HMGA2* and *MED12* alterations frequently coexist in UFs [43].

Although alterations in *MED12* and *HMGA2* have been postulated as the initial insult leading to unregulated cell growth, and there is evidence that such alterations support leiomyoma stem-cell self-renewal and cell proliferation, it is unclear whether these genetic alterations cause the transformation of a myometrial stem cell or simply support already existing leiomyoma stem-progenitor cells.

4.3 Hereditary leiomyomatosis and renal cell carcinoma

Most cases of uterine myomas are sporadic in nature; however, there are a few rare familial disorders that are accompanied by the development of uterine fibroids through genetic disorders. Hereditary leiomyomatosis and renal cell carcinoma are autosomal dominant syndromes with both cutaneous and uterine leiomyomas [44]. The risk of renal cell carcinoma and that of leiomyosarcoma are increased in this syndrome. The gene involved is fumarate hydratase (*FH*), coding for an enzyme involved in Krebs cycle. FH acts as a classic tumor suppressor; thus, inactivating mutations of *FH* significantly increase the risk of fibroids in the uterus and other tissues. Mutations in *FH* are mutually exclusive to *MED12* and *HMGA2* mutations [45].

4.4 The Alport syndrome-diffuse leiomyomatosis association

The Alport syndrome-diffuse leiomyomatosis association can be defined as a hereditary disease of type IV collagen combining features of Alport syndrome (hematuric nephropathy, deafness, and ocular abnormalities) and diffuse leiomyomatosis of the respiratory, gastrointestinal, and genitourinary tracts. The disease is caused by mutations of both the *COL4A5* and *COL4A6* genes [46].

Other recurrent genetic aberrations and chromosomal rearrangements have been identified in sporadic fibroids, such as trisomy of chromosome 12, deletions in 7q, monosomy of chromosome 22, and RAD51 gene (a DNA repair protein), among others [10, 11]. These alterations might have a common origin through a single genomic event that results in multiple chromosomal breaks and random reassembly (the so-called chromothripsis). It has been proposed that tumorigenesis occurs when tissue-specific tumor-promoting changes are formed through these events [11].

Although the aforementioned cytogenetic alterations are thought to start tumorigenesis *via* clonal proliferation, they are considered insufficient for tumor development. Therefore, alterations in several complex signaling pathways have been postulated to play an additional role in the pathogenesis of UFs.

5. Signaling pathways involved in myoma growth and development

Several complicated cellular processes, involving different signaling pathways, are thought to play a pivotal role in the pathogenesis of UFs. Currently available knowledge has identified that several of these pathways converge/interconnect/overlap in a summative way; they can act as signal integrators and incorporate inputs from other molecular pathways. This "crosstalk" between signaling pathways makes the understanding of myoma biology, and the development of targeted therapies even more difficult. The physiology and detailed description of these pathways are beyond the scope of this chapter; however, they have been well described elsewhere [47, 48].

5.1 Receptor tyrosine kinases

Receptor tyrosine kinases (RTKs) are cell-surface growth factor receptors. Generally, when growth factors bind to RTK, receptor phosphorylation (activation) leads to downstream activation of several pathways. Therefore, RTKs are important regulators of important cellular processes, such as differentiation, proliferation, and survival. There is a growing body of evidence for the role of RTKs in pathophysiology of UFs, mediating cell-to-cell interactions, and the development of an adequate tumoral microenvironment by increasing expression of the RTK downstream effectors: the mitogen-activated protein kinase/extracellular signal-regulated kinase (MAPK/ERK) and phosphoinositide 3-kinase/protein kinase B/mammalian target of rapamycin (PI3K/Akt/mTOR pathways) [47, 48]. Interestingly, previous data show that RTKs are also intermediate factors for sex steroid effects since estrogens upregulate RTKs, suggesting a crosstalk between both pathways in UFs [49–51].

5.2 MAPK/ERK pathway

The MAPK/ERK pathway (also known as the Ras/Raf/MEK/ERK pathway) is a chain of proteins that communicate signals from surface-cell receptors to the DNA in the nucleus. This pathway regulates several critical cell processes, such as cell proliferation, survival, and apoptosis. They included several subfamilies, such as extracellular signal-regulated kinases (ERKs), c-Jun N-terminal kinases (JNKs), and p38 mitogen-activated protein kinases (p38 MAPK), which have been linked to leiomyoma biology [47]. The binding of growth factors to their receptors (RTKs) leads to a cascade of molecular events that include sequential phosphorylation (activation) of Ras, Raf, MEK, and ERK proteins. In turn, ERK activates several transcription factors. This pathway has been shown to be upregulated in UFs. Moreover, it has complex and bidirectional interaction with steroid hormone-induced signals. For example, estrogen can activate this pathway through G-protein-coupled receptors and growth factors can modulate the response to steroids of MAPK/ERK through effects of MAPK/ERK on transcriptional activity of steroid receptors [47].

5.3 PI3K/Akt/mTOR pathway

The phosphoinositide 3-kinase (PI3K)/protein kinase B (Akt)/mammalian target of rapamycin (mTOR) pathway is another RTK-ligand activated intracellular signaling pathway important in regulating the cell cycle. Therefore, it is directly related to cellular quiescence, proliferation, and longevity. In addition to RTK-ligand binding,

PI3K can be activated by G-protein-coupled receptors and membrane-bound steroid receptors. To date, several studies have demonstrated aberrant PI3K/Akt/mTOR signaling in UFs [47].

5.4 Smad protein signaling

Smads are intracellular proteins that transmit signals from several cell membrane receptors to the nucleus. They are the main signal transducers for receptors of the TGF-β superfamily, including Activin-A, which are critically important for regulating cell development and growth [52]. In vertebrates, eight Smads have been identified and named Smad1 to Smad8 and they are divided in three distinct subtypes: receptor-regulated Smads (R-Smads), common partner Smads (Co-Smads), and inhibitory Smads (I-Smads). Smads exert their function by forming heterotrimers of two R-Smads and one Co-Smad that act as a transcription factor. Smad4 is the only Co-Smad described in humans. Upon ligand binding to Smad-coupled receptors, two R-Smads are phosphorylated and then heterotrimerize with one common Co-Smad (Smad4). The resulting complex translocates to the nucleus to act as a transcription factor for target genes [52]. There is evidence that UFs demonstrate aberrant Smad signaling, and that several molecules with a pivotal role in leiomyoma pathophysiology, including TGF-β, Activin-A, and myostatin, converge on Smads to regulate cellular proliferation and ECM formation at the transcriptional level [47, 52].

5.5 Wnt/β-catenin pathway

The wingless-type integration site (Wnt) family are a group of signal transduction pathways involved in several cellular functions, such as cell proliferation and differentiation, apoptosis, cell migration, and stem cell maintenance in adults. β-Catenin is a dual protein involved in the regulation and coordination of cell-cell adhesion and gene transcription. β-Catenin acts as an intracellular signal transducer in the Wnt signaling pathway [53].

Wingless-type proteins function as ligands and bind to specific receptors. When Wnt binds to its receptor, a stable β-catenin detaches from the β-catenin destruction complex and is free to translocate to the nucleus to alter gene transcription by acting as a transcriptional coactivator (the so-called canonical Wnt pathway). However, in the absence of Wnt activation, the unstable β-catenin binds to the protein destruction complex and is degraded through ubiquitination [53].

The activation of canonical Wnt pathway (β-catenin-dependent) stimulates the differentiation of resting fibroblasts into myofibroblasts and has a key role in fibrotic processes, such as myoma development [54]. In a recent article, El Sabeh et al. [53] reviewed the role of Wnt/β-catenin signaling pathway in uterine leiomyoma biology. Interestingly, evidence suggests that *MED12* mutations, which seem to drive fibroid formation (see above), are implicated in the regulation of the Wnt/β-catenin pathway. It was shown that β-catenin targeted the *MED12* to activate transcription. Moreover, the inhibition of the β-catenin/*MED12* interaction suppressed β-catenin activation in response to Wnt signaling [39]. Since *MED12* was shown to be essential for canonical Wnt signaling and *MED12* limits β-catenin-dependent growth during mouse embryonic development, it has been postulated that *MED12* mutations resulting in absent or defective *MED12* can lead to a β-catenin pathway-dependent growth [53]. Indeed, fibroids with *MED12* mutations have increased levels of Wnt4 ligand compared with those without these mutations [38]. Similarly, in a recent study using an immortalized human uterine myometrial smooth muscle cell line, the overexpression of mutant *MED12* resulted in increased expression of Wnt4 and β-catenin when compared to the cells with the overexpression of wild-type *MED12* [55]. Likewise, estrogen and the interaction of Wnt4/β-catenin pathway along with TGF-β might explain the enhanced growth observed in fibroids with *MED12* mutations [4]. Furthermore, it has been shown that TGF-β activates canonical (β-catenin-dependent) Wnt signaling and that activation of Wnt canonical signaling is required for TGF-β-mediated fibrosis [54]. In this context, Wnt pathway could provide a putative mechanism by which myometrial stem cells stimulate transformation into TICs.

As previously described, paracrine activation of the Wnt/β-catenin pathway, mediated by estrogen and progesterone, induces the nuclear translocation of β-catenin in leiomyoma stem cells [19], leading to the expression of genes with a critical role in UFs growth and development. Therefore, it has been accepted that sex steroid-induced proliferation in UFs is modulated, at least in part, through Wnt expression by mature cells and its paracrine response to β-catenin signaling in leiomyoma stem cells.

In addition, Wnt/β-catenin pathway has several crosstalks with other signaling pathways involved in UFs biology, such as PI3K/Akt/mTOR, Ras/Raf/MEK/ERK, insulin-like growth factor (IGF), and sex steroid pathways [53].

5.6 Other pathways

Aberrations in other pathways have been described in UFs, such as peroxisome proliferator-activated receptors (PPARs) and retinoic acid signaling pathways [47, 48]. Briefly, both pathways are involved in cell growth, development, and differentiation by binding nuclear receptors and finally regulating gene transcription. Interestingly, retinoic acid receptors (RARs and RXRs) act as heterodimers for several nuclear receptors, including vitamin D receptor (VDR), while PPARs act as a thyroid hormone receptor [47]. PPARs form heterodimers with RXRs to regulate gene transcription. Interestingly, retinoids might be linked to ethnic heterogeneity observed in UFs since black women have different expression profiles for RARs and RXRs compared with white women [56]. There is evidence that both pathways have an inhibitory role in leiomyoma cell proliferation. Of note, peroxisome proliferator-activated receptor gamma (PPARγ) stimulation leads to inhibition of estrogen-mediated gene expression [47].

In summary, molecular events in myoma biology are regulated through a complex network of interconnected and convergent, intracellular, extracellular, and intercellular pathways. Each pathway does not work on its own but it is a complicated network of molecular processes, although several signal transduction pathways converge into a final pathway.

6. Epigenetic modulation in myoma development

Epigenetics is defined as all heritable changes in gene expression (phenotype) that are not coded in the DNA sequence. Therefore, these changes are mediated by altered gene expression [41]. Unlike genetic changes, epigenetic changes are reversible and do not change the DNA sequence, but they can change how the DNA sequence is "read." Epigenetic changes affect gene expression by silencing (switching off), switching on, and stabilizing genes. Environment and behaviors, such as diet and exercise, can result in epigenetic changes. Epigenetic changes affect gene expression in different ways. In humans, three main epigenetic mechanisms play a role in modulating gene expression in fibroid formation:

6.1 DNA methylation and demethylation

DNA methyltransferases (DNMTs) are enzymes that catalyze the transfer of a methyl group to DNA. Typically, methylation in the promoter region is associated with suppression of gene expression. By contrast, demethylation tends to activate gene transcription [57]. Li et al. [58] found global DNA hypomethylation and decreased expression of DNMTs (DNMT3A and DMT3B) in uterine fibroids when compared to the adjacent myometrium, suggesting an epigenetic mechanism in leiomyoma development. A potential link between estrogen receptor-α gene hypomethylation and uterine fibroid formation has also been postulated [59]. Other studies have investigated the role of DNA hypermethylation in silencing tumor suppressor genes in the pathophysiology of uterine fibroids [60, 61]. Navarro et al. [61] found 55 genes with differential promoter methylation and concomitant differences in messenger RNA (mRNA) expression in uterine leiomyoma versus normal myometrium. Eighty percent of the identified genes showed an inverse relationship between DNA methylation status and mRNA expression in uterine leiomyoma tissues, and most genes (62%) displayed hypermethylation associated with gene silencing. Interestingly, they found hypermethylation, mRNA repression, and protein expression of known tumor suppressor genes in uterine leiomyomas, suggesting a possible functional role of promoter DNA methylation-mediated gene silencing in the pathogenesis of UFs [61].

6.2 Histone modification

Histone modification is the second most important epigenetic factor that has a critical role in the regulation of gene expression. Histones are proteins that act as spools around which DNA winds to create structural units called nucleosomes. Histones prevent DNA from becoming tangled and protect it from DNA damage. Histones can be modified in many ways in their N-terminal tail, including acetylation, phosphorylation, and methylation, among others. Histone methylation can determine either activation or repression of gene transcription; instead, histone acetylation determines gene activation [17]. Wei et al. [62] studied the histone deacetylase 6 (HDAC6) expression and its pathogenic role in uterine leiomyoma development. They found a regular pattern of increasing HDCA6 and estrogen receptor-α-gene expression in leiomyoma samples.

6.3 Noncoding RNA (MicroRNA)

MicroRNA (miRNA) are a novel class of small nonprotein coding, single-stranded RNAs that regulate a high number of biological processes and their related pathways, such as gene expression via gene silencing with either translational repression or degradation of mRNAs. However, more recent studies have demonstrated that some miRNAs can upregulate target genes by directly binding to their promoter [57]. Current research has proposed the role of alterations in miRNA levels in tumorigenesis. In a recent comprehensive review by Ciebiera et al. [63], the current knowledge about the role of different miRNA families in the biology of UFs is summarized. In this paper, the authors provide updated information about microRNA families and their predicted target genes that are significantly dysregulated in uterine leiomyomas compared with normal myometrium. This dysregulation affects several leiomyoma-involved signaling pathways, including MAPK/ERK, Wnt, janus kinase (JAK)-signal transducer and activator of transcription (STAT), and TGF-β [57]. The implications of such alterations affect several processes, such as tumor senescence, angiogenesis, inflammation, ECM accumulation, cell proliferation, and apoptosis [63].

Peng et al. [64] demonstrated the interaction between HMGA2 and lethal-7 (let-7) miRNAs. The repression of HMGA2 *via* let-7 s inhibited cellular proliferation *in vitro*. In the same report, microRNA profiling analysis revealed that let-7 s were significantly dysregulated in uterine leiomyomas: high in small leiomyomas (<3 cm) and lower in large leiomyomas (>10 cm). The authors hypothesized that Let-7-mediated repression of HMGA2 mechanism can be an important molecular event in leiomyoma growth.

The microRNA-21 (miR-21) family has been implicated in excessive ECM formation by stopping the Smad7 protein, an inhibitory Smad that inhibits TGF-β pathway [48]. Furthermore, the expression of transforming growth factor beta receptor 2 (TGFβR2) is the target of miR-21 in UFs, so it may mediate its biological activities by binding to TGF-β receptors [63].

The importance of the miR-29 family is one of the best known in UFs since the members of this family target several ECM-related genes. The overexpression of miR-29 s decreases the production of ECM compounds, and its expression is lower in UFs compared to normal myometrium. Interestingly, several observations have confirmed that sex steroids can downregulate miR-29 s and, as a result, upregulate collagen expression [65, 66].

A detailed description of miRNA families and their biological actions involved in UFs pathophysiology is beyond the scope of this chapter and can be found elsewhere [63, 67].

7. Growth factors

Growth factors (GFs) are proteins or peptides, produced locally by smooth muscle cells and fibroblasts and secreted into extracellular space, that take part in several cellular events, like proliferation, growth, ECM synthesis, and angiogenesis, important for leiomyoma growth [68]. GFs act over short distances either in an autocrine and/or paracrine manner and exert most of their effects on target cells by interacting with specific cell-surface receptors, with subsequent signaling transmission *via* signal transduction systems in the cell [28, 30]. Therefore, overexpression of either GFs or their receptors plays an important role in tumorigenesis. Aberration of several growth factors and their receptors or signaling pathways has been implicated in myoma pathophysiology, such as TGF-β, Activin-A, myostatin, epidermal growth factor (EGF), heparin-binding EGF (HB-EGF), platelet-derived growth factor (PDGF), insulin-like growth factor (IGF), vascular endothelial growth factor (VEGF), fibroblast growth factor 1 (FGF-1), and fibroblast growth factor 2 (FGF-2) [68]. All the above-cited GFs are ligands of RTKs and activate two critical signaling cascades such as MAPK/ERK and PI3K/Akt/mTOR pathways [48]. On the other hand, members of the TGF-β superfamily (Activin-A and myostatin) act through serine/threonine kinase receptors/Smad pathway [30], whereas TGF-β is able to activate both MAPK/ERK and serine/threonine kinase receptors/Smad pathway [17]. In this chapter, we will discuss the most researched topics and those considered the most relevant for myoma development.

7.1 Transforming growth factor-β (TGF-β)

Transforming growth factor-β are peptides that regulate ECM production as well as cell growth and differentiation and it has three different isoforms (TGF-β1, transforming growth factor-β2 (TGF-β2), and TGF-β3). It is produced by many cell types, including macrophages and myofibroblasts. TGF-β signaling has been found to be involved in diseases with abnormal ECM production and fibrosis development and there is a growing body of evidence for a role of abnormal TGF-β signaling pathways in UFs [69, 70]. Moreover, expression of TGF-β is stimulated by the Wnt/β-catenin pathway, and several studies have demonstrated a crosstalk between Wnt/β-catenin and TGF-β pathways [5, 37, 53, 54]. TGF-β shows bimodal effects on cell proliferation, induces elevated production of ECM-related genes, and decreases production of ECM degradation-related genes [17]. In addition, it can either inhibit or stimulate the proliferation of human smooth muscle cells in a dose-dependent manner. At low concentrations, TGF-β induces cell proliferation by stimulating autocrine PDGF secretion, whereas it induces the opposite effect at higher concentrations *via* down-regulation of the PDGF receptor and by direct inhibition [17, 30]. Interestingly, the most studied pathway of myofibroblast formation is TGF-β1-dependent differentiation from fibroblasts [71]. TGF-β is induced by mechanical tension and induced α-SMA expression. The expression of ECM proteins, fibronectin and fibromodulin (a collagen-binding protein), is also stimulated by TGF-β [70]. It has been shown that TGF-β receptor type 2 and 1(TGFβR2 and TGFβR1, respectively) expression is elevated in leiomyoma compared to myometrium [68]. The most common isoform found in mesenchymal cells is TGF-β3, and studies have shown that the TGF-β3 level is three-to fivefold increased in fibroids as compared with normal myometrium [69]. Moreover, it has been shown that TGF-β3 induces collagen and versican expression in leiomyoma cells and directly stimulates myometrial and leiomyoma cell proliferation [68, 70]. Although most studies on the role of TGF-β in UFs pathophysiology have focused on its role in fibrosis and ECM production, TGF-β is also related to UFs pathogenesis through its angiogenic effects [72].

From the clinical point of view, TGF-β3 regulation of bone morphogenetic proteins (BMPs), another ligand member of the TGF-β family, has been implicated in myoma-related symptoms, such as defective endometrial decidualization, impairment of endometrial receptivity, infertility, and excessive uterine bleeding due to suppression of the expression of local anticoagulant factors (such as plasminogen inhibitor activator 1, antithrombin III, and thrombomodulin) [37, 73]. TGF-β1 and TGF-β3 are considered as key players in excessive ECM accumulation and fibrosis observed in UFs, and both molecules exert their functions, such as myofibroblastic transformation, ECM remodeling, regulation of the inflammatory response and fibrosis promotion, at least in part, through activation of the MAPK/ERK and Smad 2/3 signaling pathways [17, 68].

7.2 Activin-A

Activin-A, a growth factor member of the TGF-β superfamily, has been proven to have an inflammatory and profibrotic role *via* binding to type II (activin receptor type IIA (ActRIIA), activin receptor type IIB (ActRIIB)) and type I (type I activin receptor (ActRIB), activin receptor-like kinase 4 or ALK4) [25, 68]. Activin-A has been shown to be more highly expressed in leiomyomas than normal myometrium, whereas the levels of its receptors (ActRIIA, ActRIIB, ALK4) remain unchanged [68].

A recent review postulates that Activin-A could be produced by the endometrium and myometrium as a response to physiological inflammation processes such as ovulation, menstruation, or parturition and that it can exert its actions by an autocrine/paracrine mechanism [25]. Other published study by the same authors confirmed the presence of Activin-A positive macrophages inside uterine leiomyoma tissue, demonstrating another source of Activin-A in UFs [22]. In addition, *in vitro* studies have shown that stimulation of primary myometrial and leiomyoma cells with TNF-α results in increased mRNA expression levels of Activin-A in these cells. Besides, it has been shown that local production of Activin-A by myometrial and endometrial cells favors the macrophage proinflammatory phenotype *via* positive feedback mechanism and that such mechanism could support the maintenance of an inflammatory environment inside the leiomyoma tissue [22, 25]. It has been hypothesized that Activin-A plays a central role in coordinating inflammation and myofibroblastic transition in myoma development and growth. Activin-A increases mRNA levels of several ECM components, including type I collagen, fibronectin, and versican, in leiomyomas compared to adjacent myometrium. Furthermore, Activin-A activates Smad 2/3 signaling pathway regulating gene transcription and contributing to fibrosis. Like TGF-β, Activin-A may also activate non-Smad pathways [25, 52].

7.3 Fibroblast growth factors

Two members of the FGF family have been implicated in myoma biology, particularly inducing angiogenesis. FGF-1, also known as acidic fibroblast growth factor (aFGF), and FGF-2, also known as basic fibroblast growth factor (bFGF) [30, 68]. Leiomyomas show an increased protein expression of both FGF-1 and FGF-2 compared with normal myometrium. Of note, FGF-2 was primarily bound to the ECM of myometrium and fibroids. This observation suggests that the enhanced growth of leiomyomas may be due, in part, to the presence of large amounts of FGF-2 that are stored in the ECM of these tumors [68]. There is evidence that VEGF acts in synergy with FGFs and can release bFGF from the ECM [41]. Furthermore, FGF receptor 1 (FGFR-1) and 2 (FGFR-2) expressions are increased in leiomyoma compared with adjacent myometrium. Interestingly, FGFR-1 expression is suppressed in early luteal phase in normal women, but not in women with leiomyoma-related bleeding [74]. These findings support the role of the FGF-2 ligand-receptor system in the pathogenesis of leiomyoma-related bleeding. Interestingly, despite their higher concentration, leiomyoma cells are less responsive to FGF-2 mitogenic effect compared to normal myometrial cells [68].

8. Endocrine-disrupting chemicals and fibroids

Endocrine-disrupting chemicals (EDCs) are chemicals that intervene with the endocrine system and may lead to reproductive, immune, and neurological adverse effects. Environmental exposure during critical periods of development alters the programming of normal physiologic responses, therefore, causing the rate of development of the disease to increase later in life, also known as developmental programming [10, 75]. Interaction of EDCs with nuclear receptors can change hormone function by mimicking hormone function, blocking the endogenous hormone from binding, or interfering with the production or regulation of hormones and/or their receptors. An individual EDC can interact with more than one receptor, and several EDCs can interact with the same receptor, highlighting the complex response to environmental EDC exposure [10]. Uterine development may be a particularly sensitive window to environmental exposures, as some perinatal EDC exposures have been shown to increase tumorigenesis in both experimental and human epidemiologic studies. There is a positive association between developmental diethylstilbestrol (DES) and UFs risk [75]. In addition, perinatal exposure to genistein and DES has shown to increase the penetrance and growth of UFs in animal studies [75]. The mechanisms by which EDC exposures may increase tumorigenesis are still being elucidated, but DNA instability, epigenetic mechanisms, reprogramming of the developing uterus estrogen-responsive gene expression, and stem-cell disruption that could change uterine sensitivity to steroid hormones in adulthood are emergent hypothesis [10, 75].

9. Extracellular matrix in uterine fibroids

It is universally accepted that a myriad of chemical signaling molecules has been identified in UFs and that sex hormones orchestrate the complex systems leading to fibroid development. However, these chemical and hormonal signals are only a part of the biological mechanism of myoma development, and these signals alone do not fully account for fibroid development and growth.

Excessive ECM accumulation is considered critical for myoma development and appears to play a crucial role in the formation of the bulky and stiff structure, and their associated symptoms such as excessive uterine bleeding and pelvic pain or pressure [6]. This accumulative process is due to an imbalance between synthesis and dissolution.

Most of the ECM components are secreted by fibroblasts and myofibroblasts; it has been suggested that both quantity and topology of the ECM are altered in UFs compared with the myometrium [6, 76]. Current knowledge supports the fact that the stiffness of fibroid tissue has a direct effect on the growth of the tumor through the induction of fibrosis. Fibrosis has two characteristics: (I) resistance to apoptosis leading to the persistence of fibroid cells and (II) secretion of collagen and other components of the ECM such as proteoglycans (PGs) by those cells leading to abundant disposition of highly crosslinked, disoriented, and often widely dispersed collagen fibrils [77].

In UFs, ECM accumulation is affected by growth factors (TGF-β, Activin-A, and PDGF), cytokines (TNF-α), steroid hormones (estrogen and progesterone), and miRNAs [6]. Furthermore, ECM serves as a reservoir for those growth factors and cytokines and often activation of these factors occurs in the ECM. In addition to growth factors' sequestration, excessive ECM contributes to initiate solid-state signaling [77].

Solid-state signaling, also called mechanotransduction, occurs when mechanical stress, such as osmotic pressure, shear stress, surface tension, and tensional forces, triggered by the fibroid growth, is converted to biochemical cell signals [76, 77]. Mechanotransduction is reported to have a significant role in both embryogenesis and tumorigenesis by regulating signaling pathways and gene expression [76]. The ECM and the cell communicate with each other and adapt to mechanical stimuli by an ongoing bidirectional process known as dynamic reciprocity. This process is facilitated with the help of specialized molecules such as ion channels, surface receptors, integrins, and the cytoskeleton [76, 77]. The activation of downstream mechanical signaling pathways can alter gene expression, leading to changes in ECM density, composition, and organization that ultimately affect cell shape and contractility. Mechanical signaling appears to play a crucial role in cell adhesion, migration, proliferation, and survival as well as inflammation and fibrosis [6]. Interestingly, it has been suggested that mechanotransduction system would be able to transfer signal faster than the diffusion-based system [77].

Mechanotransduction occurs at the sites of focal adhesions where heterodimeric integrins (α and β) serve as a molecular bridge between ECM and intracellular molecules/cytoskeleton, acting as mechanosensors [6, 77]. Integrins, especially integrin β1, act as transmembrane adhesion receptors that couple extracellular matrix stresses to the intracellular cytoskeleton to influence their integrity and growth. Integrin β1 has been found to be overexpressed in leiomyoma cells compared to myometrial cells [76]. When activated, integrin β guides the reorganization and polymerization of the actin filaments, further generating mechanical stress. Biochemical pathways downstream of integrin aggregation include the activation of cytoplasmic tyrosine kinases, such as focal adhesion kinase (FAK), Rho family of GTPases (Rho GTPases)/Rho-associated kinases (ROCK)/ERK/p38 MAPK signaling cascade, involved in gene expression, cell cycle regulation, and ECM remodeling [6, 76–78].

The imbalance in the deposition and degradation of an abnormal and fibrotic ECM increases mechanical stress transmitted to cells [76]. An important concept is that reciprocity is an indispensable characteristic of mechanosensitive cells. Cells sense the mechanical force from a newly generated altered ECM and further activate mechanical signaling that results in altered cell behavior and ECM remodeling [76, 77]. It has been demonstrated that UFs cells respond to the increased stress by changes in the organization of the intracellular structures, fibrosis, and deposition of excess ECM.

Therefore, fibroid cells exist in a state of increased mechanical stress due to excessive ECM and fibrosis; however, they respond inadequately, with an abnormal orientation of actin fibers, abnormal collagen, angular shape, and distortion of the nuclear envelop. These findings highlight the fact that mechanical signaling is altered in UFs [77, 78].

In a recent study, Ko et al. [79] showed that primary fibroid cells expressed higher levels of β-catenin (see above) when cultured on stiffer surfaces, highlighting the biomechanical cues influencing β-catenin expression. Interestingly, β-catenin signaling occurred independently of MED12 mutations, but was instead induced by the ECM stiffness, probably through the integrin-FAK pathway [79]. While mechanotransduction has been suggested as an important signaling pathway in UFs, the interaction between mechanotransduction and Wnt/β-catenin signaling pathways in UFs is not clearly elucidated.

The normal myometrium is composed of smooth muscle cells separated by ECM. The ECM is composed of collagen, proteoglycans, glycosaminoglycans, and elastin. Several studies comparing the differences between the normal myometrium and fibroids have demonstrated differences in ECM composition [6, 17].

Collagens are the major component of ECM that contributes to the stability and maintenance of structural integrity of the tissues. In addition to their role in wound healing and fibrosis, collagens are known to regulate cell migration, proliferation, differentiation, and survival by signaling through cell-surface receptors, such as integrins. Several collagen alterations, such as abnormal fibril structure and orientation, have been identified in UFs [17, 76, 77]. Likewise, leiomyoma cells have an abnormal expression of collagen subtypes, with overexpression of type I, III, and V collagens compared to the adjacent myometrium [17, 76]. It has been demonstrated that the expression of collagen in leiomyoma cells is regulated by TGF-β [76]. Moreover,

Koohestani et al. [80] demonstrated a direct effect of ECM collagens on the proliferation of leiomyoma smooth muscle cells through interplay between the collagen matrix and the PDGF-stimulated MAPK/ERK pathway.

Proteoglycans are another important constituent of the ECM. They are composed of a protein covalently bound to negatively charged glycosaminoglycans. Proteoglycans have been recognized not only to play a part in providing shape and biomechanical strength of tissues, but also to exhibit direct and indirect cell signaling properties. PGs interact with other ECM components, such as collagen, fibronectin, laminin, growth factors (such as TGF-β), and cytokines and through these interactions have shown to have a role in cell proliferation and differentiation [76, 77].

Versican is a large chondroitin sulfate proteoglycan that plays an important role in cell migration, adhesion, proliferation, and inflammation. The expression of versican was reported to be elevated in UFs. This increase could contribute to disorganization of ECM, increased tumor bulk, and stiffness of the fibroid, which would eventually lead to increased mechanical stress [76]. It was further demonstrated that versican expression is regulated by TGF-β3 [76]. Decorin is a small dermatan sulfate proteoglycan that regulates matrix assembly by binding to fibronectin and collagen *via* its core protein whose presence has been correlated with fibroid size [77]. Available evidence suggests that UFs contain less decorin than normal myometrial tissue [6]; however, it has a modified structure in UFs compared to normal myometrium (higher molecular weight). These features of decorin could contribute to increase osmotic pressure within the fibroid tissue [77]. Since decorin acts as an antagonist of TGF-β signaling, this increased TGF-β signaling may promote fibrosis [6].

Dermatopontin is an extracellular protein that binds to decorin and is involved in the formation of collagen fibrils. The expression of dermatopontin is decreased in myoma compared to normal myometrium [17]. Interestingly, in humans, both keloids and leiomyoma show a decreased expression of dermatopontin building a molecular link between these two fibrotic conditions [17]. There is evidence that ECM accumulation in UFs is due to an imbalance between synthesis and dissolution, like disordered wound healing observed in keloid formation.

Overall, the abnormal collagen, along with excess deposition of hydrophilic proteoglycans, not only contributes to the increase in bulk of the fibroids but also contributes to their stiffness. Paradoxically, UFs can increase in volume by up to 138% in 6 months but have a low mitotic index [4]; therefore, this accelerated growth is thought to be due to changes in the regulation of ECM components rather than cell proliferation. Leiomyoma cells exist in a state of hyperosmolarity and respond to the osmotic stress by regulating the expression of osmotic stress genes. The expression of such genes is increased in UFs, demonstrating the critical role of water homeostasis and osmotic stress in increasing fibroid stiffness [76, 77].

Other factor that plays an important role in myoma growth and regression is ECM remodeling process. This process is regulated by the combined action of matrix metalloproteinases (MMPs) that are responsible for the degradation of ECM, and the tissue inhibitors of MMPs (TIMPs) that are the physiological regulators of MMPs. The available evidence suggests that a dysregulation of MMPs and TIMPs could play a critical role in the development of a more fibrous ECM in UFs. Notably, several forms of MMPs and TIMPs are expressed differentially in UFs and normal myometrium [6]. The current research suggests that MMPs participate in other physiological processes, such as cell migration, differentiation, angiogenesis, and apoptosis [6]. Moreover, they can directly or indirectly affect the functions of various cytokines that play roles in inflammation and repair processes including interferon-β (IFN-β) and TGF-β1, among others. Likewise, MMPs enable proteolytic release of several growth factors with mitogenic properties, such as FGFs and TGF-β [6]. Interestingly, TGF-β is significantly elevated in UFs, and studies have shown a TGF-β-induced fibrotic transformation of normal myometrial cells along with decrease in the expression of MMPs [6].

Moore et al. [81] investigated the interactions between human uterine leiomyoma cells and uterine leiomyoma-derived fibroblasts, and their importance in cell growth and ECM protein production using a coculture system. They showed that uterine leiomyoma-derived fibroblasts can stimulate uterine leiomyoma cell proliferation and enhance the production of ECM proteins with elevated levels of collagen type I, several growth factors, such as platelet-derived growth factor (PDGF)-A, PDGF-B, vascular endothelial growth factor (VEGF), epidermal growth factor (EGF), TGF-β1, TGF-β3, activation of receptor tyrosine kinases (RTKs) of the mentioned growth factor ligands, and TGF-β receptor signaling. These data support that leiomyoma growth may be mediated in part by autocrine and/or paracrine mechanisms and highlight the importance of interactions between fibroid tumor cells and ECM fibroblasts *in vivo* in promoting growth factor synthesis, activating signaling pathways, and then stimulating tumor cell proliferation and production of ECM proteins [81].

10. The role of hypoxia and angiogenesis in UFs biology

The exact trigger that initiates the fibrotic process in UFs remains unclear. It has been proposed that hypoxia may play a role in triggering uterine stem cells transformation into TICs [17, 28] supporting this hypothesis. Ono et al. [82] reported that myometrial stem cells were able to differentiate into mature myometrial cells only under hypoxic conditions *in vitro*, suggesting that hypoxia may be the driving force behind their growth and transformation into leiomyoma cells. It is widely accepted that tumor environment in UFs is severally hypoxic [72, 83]. Several studies have confirmed that UFs have an abnormal vasculature. UFs have less vascular density than surrounding myometrium, and this decreased vasculature likely accounts for the severe hypoxia in fibroid tissue [72]. Recent studies have shown that UF is relatively avascular, in contrast to the peri-fibroid tissue [84]. UFs are surrounded by a dense myometrial vascular network. It has been suggested that this vascular capsule region corresponds to the vascular peripheral rim seen on ultrasound [15], and to the plane of tissue dissection during myomectomy.

Normally, angiogenic process involved an interaction between the blood vessels themselves and their surrounding ECM. Ultimately, angiogenesis depends on the balance between angiogenic factors and their inhibitors [72]. To date, it is believed that the unique vascular architecture of UFs, consisting of an avascular surrounded by a well-vascularized capsule, is most likely due to an angiogenic imbalance. Intriguingly, it is well known that the expression of several angiogenic factors is dysregulated in UFs, including EGF, HB-EGF, VEGF, bFGF, PDGF, TGF-β, and adrenomedullin [72]. There are several possible explanations for the diminished fibroid vasculature despite an increased presence of angiogenic factors, including an aberrant hypoxia response, lack of response to angiogenic promoters and overexpression of angiogenic inhibitors [72].

Tissue hypoxia is a potent stimuli for angiogenesis leading to up-regulation of hypoxia-inducible factor-Iα (HIF-Iα), which drives the expression of angiogenic factors and orchestrates the tissue adaptions to hypoxia [72]. Interestingly, HIF-Iα has not been identified in UFs [85]. Therefore, although leiomyoma tissues are hypoxic, and UFs feature down-regulation of key molecular regulators of the hypoxia response. The mechanism responsible for the lack of HIF-Iα up-regulation, which underlies the aberrant hypoxic response in UFs, remains unclear. In addition, the low vascular density observed in UF seems to be the consequence of an inadequate angiogenic response due to this altered hypoxic response [72]. Remarkably, Carmeliet et al. [86] reported that the growth of HIF-Iα-deficient tumors was not retarded but accelerated, owing to decreased hypoxia-induced apoptosis and increased stress-induced proliferation. Taken together, HIF-Iα down-regulation may explain the diminished vasculature and the continuous growth in spite of this.

On the other hand, the lack of response to angiogenic promoters could be attributed to genetic aberrations or abnormal DNA methylation observed in UFs [60]. Alternatively, an anti-angiogenic gene expression profile has been shown in UFs compared with adjacent myometrium [87].

It has been suggested that the vascularized capsule surrounding the avascular fibroid may be due to the stimulatory effects of angiogenic factor secretion by the tumor on the surrounding normal myometrium. Interestingly, Wei et al. [88] described a VEGF concentration gradient in the fibroid, with a steady increase in VEGF expression from the central zone to the periphery of the fibroid. The increased angiogenesis and vascular density observed in the normal myometrium surrounding the fibroid may account for menorrhagia in women with UFs and their tendency to bleed during myomectomy [72].

Other vascular abnormalities have been described in UFs, such as lack of smooth muscle cells and arterial spiraling when compared to normal myometrium, suggesting a vascular maturation defect. In addition, the angiogenic environment within the tumor may also suppress vessel maturation [72].

11. Vitamin D and its role in myoma biology

Vitamin D is a group of fat-soluble secosteroids (a steroid molecule with one ring open). In human biology, the most important compound in this group is vitamin D3 (cholecalciferol). Vitamin D3 is obtained from sunlight and dietary sources. By itself vitamin D3 is inactive. It is converted to its active form by two hydroxylations: the first in the liver, by the enzymes of the cytochrome P450 superfamily, CYP2R1 or CYP27A1, to form 25-hydroxycholecalciferol (calcifediol, 25-OH vitamin D3). The second hydroxylation occurs mainly in the kidney through the action of the CYP27B1 to convert 25-OH vitamin D3 into 1,25-dihydroxycholecalciferol (calcitriol, 1,25-OH2 vitamin D3), the active form of vitamin D3 [89, 90]. On the other hand, the enzyme CYP24A1 catalyzes hydroxylation reactions that lead to 1,25-OH2 vitamin D3 degradation [91].

Calcitriol acts a lipid-soluble hormone and exerts its biological actions by the activation of VDR in the nucleus. Once VDR is activated, it forms a heterodimer complex with the RXR (a retinoic acid receptor, see above). This heterodimer complex then binds to specific target DNA sequence known as the vitamin D response elements (VDREs) to modulate the expression of target genes, involved in the regulation of cell proliferation, differentiation, angiogenesis, DNA repair, and apoptosis [90]. In addition, calcitriol can bind other cell-surface receptors through second messenger pathways, exerting nongenomic actions [89, 90].

Several studies have found an association between vitamin D deficiency and the increased risk of developing UFs. It is well known that African-American women are at increased risk of developing UFs, and studies have revealed that black females have lower serum levels of vitamin D as compared with white females [89]. Moreover, an inverse relationship between vitamin D serum levels and severity of UFs has been described in this population [92]. Therefore, it can be hypothesized that these factors could lead to a loss of vitamin D functions that could explain, at least in part, why African-American females have increased incidence of UFs compared with other ethnic groups [89]. To further support this hypothesis, genomic studies have demonstrated several ethnic-related nucleotide polymorphisms, in VDR and different genes involved in vitamin D metabolism and its serum concentration, to be associated with UFs [89, 93].

In UFs, vitamin D3 inhibits the growth of both leiomyoma and myometrial cells in a concentration-dependent manner, and its serum concentration is inversely correlated with UFs size. Vitamin D3 acts an antifibrotic factor through inhibition of TGF-β3-induced fibrosis in leiomyoma cells [89, 94]. Moreover, *in vitro* studies have demonstrated that vitamin D3 also inhibits proliferation and induces apoptosis in cultured myoma cells through the downregulation of several genes involved in cell cycle regulation, and by suppression of both expression and activity of catechol-O-methyltransferase (COMT), an enzyme that modulates the biological effects of estrogens and plays a role in myoma formation [95]. Additionally, vitamin D3 suppresses the action of MMP, increases VDR and TIMPs, reduces the expression of ECM proteins, and downregulates sex hormone receptors and their coactivators, in a concentration-dependent manner [89, 96, 97].

There is evidence that UFs express reduced levels of VDR compared with myometrium, and that leiomyoma tissues showed inverse correlation between the upregulated estrogen and progesterone receptor and VDR levels [90]. A recent study by Othman et al. [91] evaluated tissue levels of active vitamin D and the expression of CYP27B1 and CYP24A1 in UFs [91]. The authors confirmed that leiomyoma cells not only contain lower level of vitamin D3 compared to myometrium, but also that uterine tissue expresses extrarenal CYP27B1. Therefore, these findings confirm that both myoma or normal myometrium tissues can produce their own active vitamin D3, and that such locally produced vitamin D3 modulates cell functions through paracrine/autocrine action. In the same study, the authors found that CYP24A1 was upregulated in UFs [91]. This mechanism not only enables UFs to degrade vitamin D3 and suppress its antitumor effects, but also to sustain a tumor microenvironment of hypovitaminosis D.

In summary, physiological actions of vitamin D are driven by the regulation of multiple cellular pathways, including proliferation, apoptosis, DNA repair, ECM deposition, and signaling. Its action in UFs cells is strictly correlated with the ability of vitamin D to control VDR expression. Moreover, dysregulation of vitamin D metabolizing enzymes observed in UFs could locally regulate vitamin D action.

In addition to its antiestrogenic/antiprogesteronic effect, VDR activation is able to suppress other relevant signaling cascades in myoma biology, such as Wnt/β-catenin, mTOR, and TGF-β pathways [47, 48, 98, 99].

12. Ovarian steroid hormones and pathogenesis of uterine fibroids

The pivotal role of ovarian steroid hormones in the pathogenesis of uterine fibroids is supported by epidemiological, clinical, and experimental evidence [100]. The fact that fibroids occur during the reproductive years and regress after menopause indicates a growth dependent on ovarian hormones [100]. Although there is no evidence of abnormal levels of circulating sex steroids in women with fibroids, tissue estrogen levels are higher in patients with UFs [101]. These findings provide some clues that tissue receptor expression, abnormal signaling, and other estrogen-related aberrations play a role in UFs development and growth.

The effects of estradiol and progesterone are interrelated and involve the mediation of receptors, transcription factors, kinase proteins, growth factors, and numerous autocrine and paracrine factors [100, 101]. As mentioned above, myometrial stem cells express very low levels of estrogen and progesterone receptors; therefore, to maintain the growth ratio, these cells require paracrine factors released from the surrounding myometrial cells expressing abundantly sex steroid receptors (crosstalk with Wnt/β-catenin) [19, 100]. Sex steroids lead to tumor expansion by stimulating a modest rate of cellular proliferation and the production of copious amount of ECM [6, 102]. Furthermore, intricate networks of postreceptor signaling can also be activated by alternative pathways that bypass the hormone-receptor complex, thus allowing hormone-like effects by nonhormonal mediators [48].

12.1 Estrogens

Estrogens are a key element of UFs pathogenesis. Estrogens elicit its physiological effects on the target cells by binding to estrogen receptors (ERs). ERs are currently classified into nuclear (classical) and membrane-bound (mERs). Nuclear ERs are subdivided in estrogen receptor alpha (ERα) and estrogen receptor beta (ERβ). On the other hand, mERs are localized at the plasma membrane and are subdivided in α, β, and G-protein-coupled estrogen receptor 1 (GPER1). GPER1 is also known as G-protein-coupled receptor 30 (GPR30). All ERs are expressed in fibroids following the differentiation of fibroid progenitor cells [47, 101, 102].

Estrogen-dependent signaling pathways can be classified as genomic and nongenomic. The genomic (transcriptional) pathway is mainly mediated by nuclear ERs. In this pathway, the estrogen-ER complex binds estrogen response elements (EREs) of DNA to regulate gene transcription. Conversely, nongenomic pathway is mainly mediated by mERs and GPER1 and works in a similar way to GFs receptors: rapidly activating downstream signaling cascades, including MAPK/ERK, PI3/Akt/mTOR and phospholipase C (PLC)/inositol trisphosphate (IP3)/calcium, among others. Furthermore, there is evidence of crosstalk between rapid estrogen signaling and GFs signaling through RTKs [101].

In addition to activation from estrogen binding, ERα is also activated by the MAPK pathway and *via* other kinases. Therefore, estrogen-bound ERα induces GFs expression, which can then stimulate the MAPK pathway and further activate ERα in an autocrine fashion. This feedback by MAPK on ERs is an example of the complexity and interconnectedness of signaling pathways in UFs [101, 102]. Interestingly, rapid activation of MAPK pathway by estrogen in primary myoma cells was related to estrogen-induced PDGF secretion and it was proposed that PDGF, alone or associated with other GFs, was the main GF involved in the proliferation response of leiomyoma cells to estrogen stimulation.

Estrogen upregulates the expression of several genes involved in UFs pathogenesis, including growth factors and their receptors (VEGF, PDGF, IGF-I, TGF-β), collagens, GPR1, and ERs [17, 101, 103].

Likewise, estrogen sensitizes the tissue to progesterone by promoting expression of progesterone receptor, providing a microenvironment in which progesterone can induce fibroid growth [100–102]. Conversely, estrogen downregulates Activin-A and myostatin expression [17]. Importantly, it has been shown that many of these processes occur only in UFs cells but not in normal myometrium; therefore, it has been postulated that this differential effect can be a contributing factor in UFs pathobiology [101].

Interestingly, it has been shown that even if estrogen downregulates EGF expression, it upregulates the expression of its receptors (epidermal growth factor receptors (EGFRs)). Interestingly, estrogen activation of GPR1 induces MMP activation and release of HB-EGF which binds and activates upregulated EGFRs. This transactivation represents an important integrator of estrogen and GF cellular signaling [101].

Other actions of estrogen include the inactivation of several tumor suppressor genes, such as p53, providing insight into tumor transformation mechanisms in UFs and how they are closely linked to estrogen signaling [17, 101].

Estrogen receptors are abundantly expressed in uterine myomas, which ensure considerable responsiveness to the circulating estrogen. Whether UFs are richer in ERs than surrounding myometrium is still debatable, with some studies showing such a difference, whereas others do not [17, 100]. However, there is an enhanced response to estrogen stimulation by fibroid cells compared to normal myometrium.

Moreover, studies have demonstrated that ethnic-related polymorphisms, involving ERs [104, 105] and elements of estrogen signaling and metabolism, such as aromatase (CYP19A1) [106, 107] and COMT [108], are related to the increased leiomyoma risk in different ethnic groups.

Uterine fibroids are exposed to estrogen not only through ovarian steroidogenesis, but also through local conversion of androgens by aromatase within the tumors themselves. Interestingly, a quantifiable increase in aromatase expression has been found in African-American women [106]. Therefore, UFs are capable of producing enough estrogen to sustain their own growth. Furthermore, UFs have remarkably levels of aromatase compared with adjacent myometrium [102].

12.2 Progesterone

Progesterone action is required for full development and proliferation of myoma cells, and available data suggest that progesterone might be the primary hormone driving the growth of UFs. Estrogen is also necessary, but not sufficient for myoma growth [102]. Ishikawa et al. [109] showed that estrogen/ERα regulates progesterone receptor expression and that estrogen alone is not a mitogen *in vivo*. These findings suggest a more permissive role for estrogen acting *via* induction of PR expression, and thereby allowing UFs responsiveness to progesterone (estrogen-progesterone crosstalk) [47].

In UFs, progesterone actions are mediated by nuclear progesterone receptors A and B (PR-A and PR-B) [47, 102]. Several studies have demonstrated increased expression of both PR-A and PR-B in UFs compared to normal myometrium, and that it seems to be even higher according to women's age and number of tumors [100]. Interestingly, an overexpression of PR-B has been found on UFs surface, suggesting that the predominant expression of PR-B in this part reveals an activated phenotype for progestational proliferation related to myoma growth [17]. Furthermore, studies have demonstrated that mitotic activity in UFs is significantly higher in secretory (progesterone-dominant) phase of the menstrual cycle [47]. Conversely, PRs expression is lower in women experiencing severe bleeding and dysmenorrhea [100]. Ligand-bound PR binds to DNA and regulates transcription of several target genes.

In addition to this transcriptional pathway, progesterone can activate rapid signaling pathways (nongenomic). Activated PRs activate MAPK/ERK signaling pathway. Moreover, it has been shown that progesterone can rapidly activate PI3/Akt pathway inducing UFs growth [110].

Progesterone influences myoma growth by the interaction with GFs (progesterone-GFs signaling crosstalk), and other genes involved in cell proliferation, including upregulation of TGF-β1, TGF-β3, EGF and expression of B-cell lymphoma 2 (Bcl-2) oncogene [17, 47, 110]. On the other hand, progesterone inhibits IGF-I, TNF-α, and decorin expression in myoma cells. Since decorin inhibits TGF-β activity, its reduced levels in leiomyoma may enhance TGF-β-mediated ECM deposition [6, 17].

Finally, there is much more to be learned in terms of how progesterone promotes proliferation, the repertoire of genes involved, and how progesterone and GFs signaling pathways crosstalk in leiomyomas.

13. Conclusions

The hallmarks of uterine fibroid development and growth are clonal expansion of an aberrant myometrial stem cell and excessive deposition of extracellular matrix.

Although alterations in MED12 and HMGA2 have been postulated as the initial insult leading to unregulated cell growth, it is unclear whether these genetic alterations cause the transformation of a myometrial stem cell or simply support already existing leiomyoma stem-progenitor cells.

Extracellular matrix acts as a reservoir of growth factors and protects them from degradation. In addition, sex steroids increase ECM production by regulating expression and activity of growth factors. These processes are tightly regulated through a complex network of interconnected signaling pathways.

We have discussed the putative role of inflammation and an abnormal hypoxia response in myoma development and the role of myofibroblasts as the central player in those aberrant processes.

Even though some cell-related events have been identified, the exact cell of origin and the exact molecular processes involved in uterine leiomyomas formation remain unknown.

Conflict of interest

The authors declare no conflict of interest.

Author details

Demetrio Larraín* and Jaime Prado
Obstetric and Gynecology Department, Minimally Invasive Surgery Unit, Clínica Santa María, Santiago, Chile

*Address all correspondence to: dlarraind@gmail.com

References

[1] Stewart EA, Cookson CL, Gandolfo RA, Schulze-Rath R. Epidemiology of uterine fibroids: A systematic review. BJOG: An International Journal of Obstetrics & Gynaecology. 2017;**124**(10):1501-1512. DOI: 10.1111/1 10.1002/gcc.20035471-0528.14640

[2] Cardozo ER, Clark AD, Banks NK, Henne MB, Stegmann BJ, Segars JH. The estimated annual cost of uterine leiomyomata in the United States. American Journal of Obstetrics and Gynecology. 2012;**206**(3):211.e1-211.e9. DOI: 10.1016/j.ajog.2011.12.002

[3] Holdsworth-Carson SJ, Zaitseva M, Vollenhoven BJ, Rogers PAW. Clonality of smooth muscle and fibroblast cell populations isolated from human fibroid and myometrial tissues. Molecular Human Reproduction. 2014;**20**(3):250-259. DOI: 10.1093/molehr/gat083

[4] Stewart EA, Laughlin-Tommaso SK, Catherino WH, Lalitkumar S, Gupta D, Vollenhoven B. Uterine fibroids. Nature Reviews Disease Primers. 2016;**2**:16043. DOI: 10.1038/nrdp.2016.43 DOI : 10.1093/molehr/gat083

[5] Bulun SE. Uterine fibroids. The New England Journal of Medicine. 2013;**369**(14):1344-1355. DOI: 10.1056/nejmcp1411029

[6] Islam MS, Ciavattini A, Petraglia F, Castellucci M, Ciarmela P. Extracellular matrix in uterine leiomyoma pathogenesis: A potential target for future therapeutics. Human Reproduction Update. 2018;**24**(1):59-85. DOI: 10.1093/humupd/dmx032

[7] Parker WH. Etiology, symptomatology, and diagnosis of uterine myomas. Fertility and Sterility. 2007;**87**(4):725-736. DOI: 10.1016/j.fertnstert.2007.01.093

[8] Lin CY, Wang CM, Chen ML, Hwang BF. The effects of exposure to air pollution on the development of uterine fibroids. International Journal of Hygiene and Environmental Health. 2019;**222**(3):549-555. DOI: 10.1016/j.ijheh.2019.02.004

[9] Ono M, Qiang W, Serna VA, Yin P, Coon JS, Navarro A, et al. Role of stem cells in human uterine leiomyoma growth. PLoS One. 2012;**7**(5):e36935. DOI: 10.1371/journal.pone.0036935

[10] Elkafas H, Qiwei Y, Al-Hendy A. Origin of uterine fibroids: Conversion of myometrial stem cells to tumor-initiating cells. Seminars in Reproductive Medicine. 2017;**35**(6):481-486. DOI: 10.1055/s-0037-1607205

[11] Mas A, Cervello I, Gil-Sanchis C, Simón C. Current understanding of somatic stem cells in leiomyoma formation. Fertility and Sterility. 2014;**102**(3):613-620. DOI: 10.1016/j.fertnstert.2014.04.051

[12] Ono M, Bulun SE, Maruyama T. Tissue-specific stem cells in the myometrium and tumor-initiating cells in leiomyoma. Biology of Reproduction. 2014;**91**(6):149. DOI: 10.1095/biolreprod.114.123794

[13] Lee M, Cheon K, Chae B, Hwang H, Kim HK, Chung YJ, et al. Analysis of MED12 mutation in multiple uterine leiomyomas in South Korean patients. International Journal of Medical Sciences. 2018;**15**(2):124-128. DOI: 10.7150/ijms.21856

[14] Peddada SD, Laughlin SK, Miner K, Guyon JP, Haneke K, Vahdat HL, et al. Growth of uterine leiomyomata among

premenopausal black and white women. Proceedings of the National Academy of Sciences of the United States of America. 2008;**105**(50):19887-19892 DPI: 10.1073/pnas.0808188105

[15] Tsiligiannis SE, Zaitseva M, Coombs PR, Shekleton P, Olshansky M, Hickey M, et al. Fibroid-associated heavy menstrual bleeding: Correlation between clinical features, doppler ultrasound assessment of vasculature, and tissue gene expression profiles. Reproductive sciences (Thousand Oaks, Calif.). 2013;**20**(4):361-370. DOI: 10.1177/1933719112459233

[16] Holdsworth-Carson SJ, Zaitseva M, Girling JE, Vollenhoven BJ, Rogers PAW. Common fibroid-associated genes are differentially expressed in phenotypically dissimilar cell populations isolated from within human fibroids and myometrium. Reproduction (Cambridge, England). 2014;**147**(5):683-692. DOI: 10.1530/rep-13-0580

[17] Islam MS, Protic O, Stortoni P, Grechi G, Lamanna P, Petraglia F, et al. Complex networks of multiple factors in the pathogenesis of uterine leiomyoma. Fertility and Sterility. 2013;**100**(1):178-193. DOI: 10.1016/j.fertnstert.2013.03.007

[18] Zhou S, Yi T, Shen K, Zhang B, Huang F, Zhao X. Hypoxia: The driving force of uterine myometrial stem cells differentiation into leiomyoma cells. Medical Hypotheses. 2011;**77**(6):985-986. DOI: 10.1016/j.mehy.2011.08.026

[19] Ono M, Yin P, Navarro A, Moravek MB, Coon JS, Druschitz SA, et al. Paracrine activation of WNT/β-catenin pathway in uterine leiomyoma stem cells promotes tumor growth. Proceedings of the National Academy of Sciences of the United States of America. 2013;**110**(42):17053-17058. DOI: 10.1073/pnas.1313650110

[20] Tanwar PS, Lee HJ, Zhang L, Zukerberg LR, Taketo MM, Rueda BR, et al. Constitutive activation of Beta-catenin in uterine stroma and smooth muscle leads to the development of mesenchymal tumors in mice. Biology of Reproduction. 2009;**81**(3):545-552. DOI: 10.1095/biolreprod.108.075648

[21] Islam MS, Catherino WH, Protic O, Janjusevic M, Gray PC, Giannubilo SR, et al. Role of activin-A and myostatin and their signaling pathway in human myometrial and leiomyoma cell function. The Journal of Clinical Endocrinology and Metabolism. 2014;**99**(5):E775-E785. DOI: 10.1210/jc.2013-2623

[22] Protic O, Toti P, Islam MS, Occhini R, Giannubilo SR, Catherino WH, et al. Possible involvement of inflammatory/reparative processes in the development of uterine fibroids. Cell and Tissue Research. 2016;**364**(2):415-427. DOI: 10.1007/s00441-015-2324-3

[23] Wynn TA. Cellular and molecular mechanisms of fibrosis. The Journal of Pathology. 2008;**214**(2):199-210. DOI: 10.1002/path.2277

[24] Hinz B, Phan SH, Thannickal VJ, Prunotto M, Desmoulière A, Varga J, et al. Recent developments in myofibroblast biology: Paradigms for connective tissue remodeling. The American Journal of Pathology. 2012;**180**(4):1340-1355. DOI: 10.1016/j.ajpath.2012.02.004

[25] Protic O, Islam MS, Greco S, Giannubilo SR, Lamanna P, Petraglia F, et al. Activin A in inflammation, tissue repair, and fibrosis: Possible role as inflammatory and fibrotic mediator of uterine fibroid development and growth. Seminars in Reproductive Medicine. 2017;**35**(6):499-509. DOI: 10.1055/s-0037-1607265

[26] Catherino WH, Leppert PC, Stenmark MH, Payson M,

Potlog-Nahari C, Nieman LK, et al. Reduced dermatopontin expression is a molecular link between uterine leiomyomas and keloids. Genes, Chromosomes & Cancer. 2004;**40**(3):204-217. DOI: 10.1002/gcc.20035

[27] Hinz B, Phan SH, Thannickal VJ, Galli A, Bochaton-Piallat ML, Gabbiani G. The myofibroblast: One function, multiple origins. The American Journal of Pathology. 2007;**170**(6):1807-1816. DOI: 10.2353/ajpath.2007.070112

[28] Chegini N. Proinflammatory and profibrotic mediators: Principal effectors of leiomyoma development as a fibrotic disorder. Seminars in Reproductive Medicine. 2010;**28**(3):180-203. DOI: 10.1055/s-0030-1251476

[29] Orciani M, Caffarini M, Biagini A, Lucarini G, Delli Carpini G, Berretta A, et al. Chronic inflammation may enhance leiomyoma development by the involvement of progenitor cells. Stem Cells International. 2018;**2018**:1716246. DOI: /10.1155/2018/1716246

[30] Ciarmela P, Islam MS, Reis FM, Gray PC, Bloise E, Petraglia F, et al. Growth factors and myometrium: Biological effects in uterine fibroid and possible clinical implications. Human Reproduction Update. 2011;**17**(6):772-790. DOI: 10.1093/humupd/dmr031

[31] Desmoulière A, Geinoz A, Gabbiani F, Gabbiani G. Transforming growth factor-beta 1 induces alpha-smooth muscle actin expression in granulation tissue myofibroblasts and in quiescent and growing cultured fibroblasts. The Journal of Cell Biology. 1993;**122**(1):103-111. DOI: 10.1083/jcb.122.1.103

[32] Vallée A, Lecarpentier Y. TGF-β in fibrosis by acting as a conductor for contractile properties of myofibroblasts. Cell & Bioscience. 2019;**9**:98. DOI: 10.1186/s13578-019-0362-3

[33] Vikhlyaeva EM, Khodzhaeva ZS, Fantschenko ND. Familial predisposition to uterine leiomyomas. International Journal of Gynaecology and Obstetrics: The Official Organ of the International Federation of Gynaecology and Obstetrics. 1995;**51**(2):127-131. DOI: 10.1016/0020-7292(95)02533-i

[34] Treloar SA, Do KA, Martin NG. Genetic influences on the age at menopause. Lancet (London, England). 1998;**352**(9134):1084-1085. DOI: 10.1016/s0140-6736(05)79753-1

[35] Levy G, Hill MJ, Beall S, Zarek SM, Segars JH, Catherino WH. Leiomyoma: Genetics, assisted reproduction, pregnancy and therapeutic advances. Journal of Assisted Reproduction and Genetics. 2012;**29**(8):703-712. DOI: 10.1007/s10815-012-9784-0

[36] Mäkinen N, Mehine M, Tolvanen J, Kaasinen E, Li Y, Lehtonen HJ, et al. MED12, the mediator complex subunit 12 gene, is mutated at high frequency in uterine leiomyomas. Science. 2011;**334**(6053):252-255. DOI: 10.1126/science.1208930

[37] Ciebiera M, Włodarczyk M, Wrzosek M, Męczekalski B, Nowicka G, Łukaszuk K, et al. Role of transforming growth factor β in uterine fibroid biology. International Journal of Molecular Sciences. 2017;**18**(11):2435. DOI: 10.3390/ijms18112435

[38] Markowski DN, Bartnitzke S, Löning T, Drieschner N, Helmke BM, Bullerdiek J. MED12 mutations in uterine fibroids--their relationship to cytogenetic subgroups. International Journal of Cancer. 2012;**131**(7):1528-1536. DOI: 10.1002/ijc.27424

[39] Kim S, Xu X, Hecht A, Boyer TG. Mediator is a transducer of Wnt/beta-catenin signaling. The Journal of Biological Chemistry. 2006;**281**(20):14066-14075. DOI: 10.1074/jbc.m602696200

[40] Al-Hendy A, Laknaur A, Diamond MP, Ismail N, Boyer TG, Halder SK. Silencing Med12 gene reduces proliferation of human leiomyoma cells mediated via Wnt/β-catenin signaling pathway. Endocrinology. 2017;**158**(3):592-603. DOI: 10.1210/en.2016-1097

[41] Laganà AS, Vergara D, Favilli A, La Rosa VL, Tinelli A, Gerli S, et al. Epigenetic and genetic landscape of uterine leiomyomas: A current view over a common gynecological disease. Archives of Gynecology and Obstetrics. 2017;**296**(5):855-867. DOI: 10.1007/s00404-017-4515-5

[42] Bertsch E, Qiang W, Zhang Q, Espona-Fiedler M, Druschitz S, Liu Y, et al. MED12 and HMGA2 mutations: Two independent genetic events in uterine leiomyoma and leiomyosarcoma. Modern Pathology. 2014;**27**(8):1144-1153. DOI: 10.1038/modpathol.2013.243

[43] Galindo LJ, Hernández-Beeftink T, Salas A, Jung Y, Reyes R, de Oca FM, et al. HMGA2 and MED12 alterations frequently co-occur in uterine leiomyomas. Gynecologic Oncology. 2018;**150**(3):562-568. DOI: 10.1016/j.ygyno.2018.07.007

[44] Schmidt LS, Linehan WM. Hereditary leiomyomatosis and renal cell carcinoma. International Journal of Nephrology and Renovascular Disease. 2014;7:253-260. DOI: 10.2147/ijnrd.s42097

[45] Mäkinen N, Kämpjärvi K, Frizzell N, Bützow R, Vahteristo P. Characterization of MED12, HMGA2, and FH alterations reveals molecular variability in uterine smooth muscle tumors. Molecular Cancer. 2017;**16**(1):101. DOI: 10.1186/s12943-017-0672-1

[46] Garcia-Torres R, Cruz D, Orozco L, Heidet L, Gubler MC. Alport syndrome and diffuse leiomyomatosis. Clinical aspects, pathology, molecular biology and extracellular matrix studies. A synthesis. Néphrologie. 2000;**21**(1):9-12

[47] Borahay MA, Al-Hendy A, Kilic GS, Boehning D. Signaling pathways in leiomyoma: Understanding pathobiology and implications for therapy. Molecular Medicine. 2015;**21**(1):242-256. DOI: 10.2119/molmed.2014.00053

[48] Cetin E, Al-Hendy A, Ciebiera M. Non-hormonal mediators of uterine fibroid growth. Current Opinion in Obstetrics & Gynecology. 2020;**32**(5):361-370. DOI: 10.1097/gco.0000000000000650

[49] Yu L, Saile K, Swartz CD, He H, Zheng X, Kissling GE, et al. Differential expression of receptor tyrosine kinases (RTKs) and IGF-I pathway activation in human uterine leiomyomas. Molecular Medicine (Cambridge, Mass.). 2008;**14**(5-6):264-275. DOI: 10.2119/2007-00101.yu

[50] Yu L, Moore AB, Dixon D. Receptor tyrosine kinases and their hormonal regulation in uterine leiomyoma. Seminars in Reproductive Medicine. 2010;**28**(3):250-259. DOI: 10.1055/s-0030-1251482

[51] Swartz CD, Afshari CA, Yu L, Hall KE, Dixon D. Estrogen-induced changes in IGF-I, Myb family and MAP kinase pathway genes in human uterine leiomyoma and normal uterine smooth muscle cell lines. Molecular Human Reproduction. 2005;**11**(6):441-450. DOI: 10.1093/molehr/gah174

[52] Derynck R, Zhang YE. Smad-dependent and Smad-independent pathways in TGF-beta family signalling. Nature. 2003;**425**(6958):577-584. DOI: 10.1038/nature02006

[53] El Sabeh M, Saha SK, Afrin S, Islam MS, Borahay MA. Wnt/β-catenin signaling pathway in uterine leiomyoma: Role in tumor biology and targeting opportunities. Molecular and Cellular Biochemistry. 2021;**476**(9):3513-3536. DOI: 10.1007/s11010-021-04174-6

[54] Akhmetshina A, Palumbo K, Dees C, Bergmann C, Venalis P, Zerr P, et al. Activation of canonical Wnt signalling is required for TGF-β-mediated fibrosis. Nature Communications. 2012;**3**:735. DOI: 10.1038/ncomms1734

[55] El Andaloussi A, Al-Hendy A, Ismail N, Boyer TG, Halder SK. Introduction of somatic mutation in MED12 induces Wnt4/β-catenin and disrupts autophagy in human uterine myometrial cell. Reproductive sciences (Thousand Oaks, Calif.). 2020;**27**(3):823-832. DOI: 10.1007/s43032-019-00084-7

[56] Wei JJ, Chiriboga L, Arslan AA, Melamed J, Yee H, Mittal K. Ethnic differences in expression of the dysregulated proteins in uterine leiomyomata. Human Reproduction (Oxford, England). 2006;**21**(1):57-67. DOI: 10.1093/humrep/dei309

[57] Styer AK, Rueda BR. The epidemiology and genetics of uterine leiomyoma. Best Practice & Research. Clinical Obstetrics & Gynaecology. 2016;**34**:3-12. DOI: 10.1016/j.bpobgyn.2015.11.018

[58] Li S, Chin CT, Richard-Davis G, Barrett JC, Mclachlan JA. DNA hypomethylation and imbalanced expression of DNA methyltransferases (DNMT1, 3A, and 3B) in human uterine leiomyoma. Gynecologic Oncology. 2003;**90**(1):123-130. DOI: 10.1016/s0090-8258(03)00194-x

[59] Asada H, Yamagata Y, Taketani T, Matsuoka A, Tamura H, Hattori N, et al. Potential link between estrogen receptor-alpha gene hypomethylation and uterine fibroid formation. Molecular Human Reproduction. 2008;**14**(9):539-545. DOI: 10.1093/molehr/gan045

[60] Yamagata Y, Maekawa R, Asada H, Taketani T, Tamura I, Tamura H, et al. Aberrant DNA methylation status in human uterine leiomyoma. Molecular Human Reproduction. 2009;**15**(4):259-267. DOI: 10.1093/molehr/gap010

[61] Navarro A, Yin P, Monsivais D, Lin SM, Du P, Wei JJ, et al. Genome-wide DNA methylation indicates silencing of tumor suppressor genes in uterine leiomyoma. PLoS One. 2012;**7**(3):e33284. DOI: 10.1371/journal.pone.0033284

[62] Wei LH, Torng PL, Hsiao SM, Jeng YM, Chen MW, Chen CA. Histone deacetylase 6 regulates estrogen receptor alpha in uterine leiomyoma. Reproductive Sciences (Thousand Oaks, Calif.). 2011;**18**(8):755-762. DOI: 10.1177/1933719111398147

[63] Ciebiera M, Włodarczyk M, Zgliczyński S, Łoziński T, Walczak K, Czekierdowski A. The role of miRNA and related pathways in pathophysiology of uterine fibroids-from bench to bedside. International Journal of Molecular Sciences. 2020;**21**(8):3016. DOI: 10.3390/ijms21083016

[64] Peng Y, Laser J, Shi G, Mittal K, Melamed J, Lee P, et al. Antiproliferative effects by Let-7 repression of high-mobility group A2 in uterine leiomyoma. Molecular Cancer Research: MCR. 2008;**6**(4):663-673. DOI: 10.1158/1541-7786.MCR-07-0370

[65] Qiang W, Liu Z, Serna VA, Druschitz SA, Liu Y, Espona-Fiedler M, et al. Down-regulation of miR-29b is essential for pathogenesis of uterine leiomyoma. Endocrinology. 2014;**155**(3):663-669. DOI: 10.1210/en.2013-1763

[66] Marsh EE, Steinberg ML, Parker JB, Wu J, Chakravarti D, Bulun SE. Decreased expression of microRNA-29 family in leiomyoma contributes to increased major fibrillar collagen production. Fertility and Sterility. 2016;**106**(3):766-772. DOI: 10.1016/j.fertnstert.2016.05.001

[67] Karmon AE, Cardozo ER, Rueda BR, Styer AK. MicroRNAs in the development and pathobiology of uterine leiomyomata: Does evidence support future strategies for clinical intervention? Human Reproduction Update. 2014;**20**(5):670-687. DOI: 10.1093/humupd/dmu017

[68] Islam MS, Greco S, Janjusevic M, Ciavattini A, Giannubilo SR, D'Adderio A, et al. Growth factors and pathogenesis. Best Practice & Research. Clinical Obstetrics & Gynaecology. 2016;**34**:25-36. DOI: 10.1016/j.bpobgyn.2015.08.018

[69] Lee BS, Nowak RA. Human leiomyoma smooth muscle cells show increased expression of transforming growth factor-beta 3 (TGF beta 3) and altered responses to the antiproliferative effects of TGF beta. The Journal of Clinical Endocrinology and Metabolism. 2001;**86**(2):913-920

[70] Arici A, Sozen I. Transforming growth factor-beta3 is expressed at high levels in leiomyoma where it stimulates fibronectin expression and cell proliferation. Fertility and Sterility. 2000;**73**(5):1006-1011

[71] Kisseleva T, Brenner DA. Mechanisms of fibrogenesis. Experimental Biology and Medicine (Maywood, N.J.). 2008;**233**(2):109-122

[72] Tal R, Segars JH. The role of angiogenic factors in fibroid pathogenesis: Potential implications for future therapy. Human Reproduction Update. 2014;**20**(2):194-216

[73] Sinclair DC, Mastroyannis A, Taylor HS. Leiomyoma simultaneously impair endometrial BMP-2-mediated decidualization and anticoagulant expression through secretion of TGF-β3. The Journal of Clinical Endocrinology and Metabolism. 2011;**96**(2):412-421

[74] Anania CA, Stewart EA, Quade BJ, Hill JA, Nowak RA. Expression of the fibroblast growth factor receptor in women with leiomyomas and abnormal uterine bleeding. Molecular Human Reproduction. 1997;**3**(8):685-691

[75] Katz TA, Yang Q, Treviño LS, Walker CL, Al-Hendy A. Endocrine-disrupting chemicals and uterine fibroids. Fertility and Sterility. 2016;**106**(4):967-977

[76] Rafique S, Segars JH, Leppert PC. Mechanical signaling and extracellular matrix in uterine fibroids. Seminars in Reproductive Medicine. 2017;**35**(6):487-493

[77] Leppert PC, Jayes FL, Segars JH. The extracellular matrix contributes to mechanotransduction in uterine fibroids. Obstetrics and Gynecology International. 2014;**2014**:783289

[78] Rogers R, Norian J, Malik M, Christman G, Abu-Asab M, Chen F, et al. Mechanical homeostasis is altered in uterine leiomyoma. American Journal of Obstetrics and Gynecology. 2008;**198**(4):474.e1-474.11

[79] Ko YA, Jamaluddin MFB, Adebayo M, Bajwa P, Scott RJ, Dharmarajan AM, et al. Extracellular matrix (ECM) activates

β-catenin signaling in uterine fibroids. Reproduction (Cambridge, England). 2018;**155**(1):61-71

[80] Koohestani F, Braundmeier AG, Mahdian A, Seo J, Bi J, Nowak RA. Extracellular matrix collagen alters cell proliferation and cell cycle progression of human uterine leiomyoma smooth muscle cells. PLoS One. 2013;**8**(9):e75844

[81] Moore AB, Yu L, Swartz CD, Zheng X, Wang L, Castro L, et al. Human uterine leiomyoma-derived fibroblasts stimulate uterine leiomyoma cell proliferation and collagen type I production, and activate RTKs and TGF beta receptor signaling in coculture. Cell Communication and Signaling (CCS). 2010;**8**:10

[82] Ono M, Maruyama T, Masuda H, Kajitani T, Nagashima T, Arase T, et al. Side population in human uterine myometrium displays phenotypic and functional characteristics of myometrial stem cells. Proceedings of the National Academy of Sciences. 2007;**104, 47**:18700-18705

[83] Mayer A, Höckel M, Wree A, Leo C, Horn LC, Vaupel P. Lack of hypoxic response in uterine leiomyomas despite severe tissue hypoxia. Cancer Research. 2008;**68**(12):4719-4726

[84] Walocha JA, Litwin JA, Miodoński AJ. Vascular system of intramural leiomyomata revealed by corrosion casting and scanning electron microscopy. Human Reproduction (Oxford, England). 2003;**18**(5):1088-1093

[85] Mayer A, Hoeckel M, von Wallbrunn A, Horn LC, Wree A, Vaupel P. HIF-mediated hypoxic response is missing in severely hypoxic uterine leiomyomas. Advances in Experimental Medicine and Biology. 2010;**662**:399-405

[86] Carmeliet P, Dor Y, Herbert JM, Fukumura D, Brusselmans K, Dewerchin M, et al. Role of HIF-1alpha in hypoxia-mediated apoptosis, cell proliferation and tumour angiogenesis. Nature. 1998;**394**(6692):485-490

[87] Weston G, Trajstman AC, Gargett CE, Manuelpillai U, Vollenhoven BJ, Rogers PAW. Fibroids display an anti-angiogenic gene expression profile when compared with adjacent myometrium. Molecular Human Reproduction. 2003;**9**(9):541-549

[88] Wei JJ, Zhang XM, Chiriboga L, Yee H, Perle MA, Mittal K. Spatial differences in biologic activity of large uterine leiomyomata. Fertility and Sterility. 2006;**85**(1):179-187

[89] Brakta S, Diamond JS, Al-Hendy A, Diamond MP, Halder SK. Role of vitamin D in uterine fibroid biology. Fertility and Sterility. 2015;**104**(3):698-706

[90] Vergara D, Catherino WH, Trojano G, Tinelli A. Vitamin D: Mechanism of action and biological effects in uterine fibroids. Nutrients. 2021;**13**(2):597

[91] Othman ER, Ahmed E, Sayed AA, Hussein M, Abdelaal II, Fetih AN, et al. Human uterine leiomyoma contains low levels of 1, 25 dihdroxyvitamin D3, and shows dysregulated expression of vitamin D metabolizing enzymes. European Journal of Obstetrics, Gynecology, and Reproductive Biology. 2018;**229**:117-122

[92] Sabry M, Halder SK, Allah ASA, Roshdy E, Rajaratnam V, Al-Hendy A. Serum vitamin D3 level inversely correlates with uterine fibroid volume in different ethnic groups: A cross-sectional observational study. International Journal of Women's Health. 2013;**5**:93-100

[93] Shahbazi S. Exploring the link between VDR rs2228570 and uterine leiomyoma in Iranian women. Egyptian Journal of Medical Human Genetics. 2016;**17**(1):115-118

[94] Halder SK, Goodwin JS, Al-Hendy A. 1,25-Dihydroxyvitamin D3 reduces TGF-beta3-induced fibrosis-related gene expression in human uterine leiomyoma cells. The Journal of Clinical Endocrinology and Metabolism. 2011;**96**(4):E754-E762

[95] Sharan C, Halder SK, Thota C, Jaleel T, Nair S, Al-Hendy A. Vitamin D inhibits proliferation of human uterine leiomyoma cells via catechol-O-methyltransferase. Fertility and Sterility. 2011;**95**(1):247-253

[96] Halder SK, Osteen KG, Al-Hendy A. 1,25-dihydroxyvitamin d3 reduces extracellular matrix-associated protein expression in human uterine fibroid cells. Biology of Reproduction. 2013;**89**(6):150

[97] Al-Hendy A, Diamond MP, El-Sohemy A, Halder SK. 1,25-dihydroxyvitamin D3 regulates expression of sex steroid receptors in human uterine fibroid cells. The Journal of Clinical Endocrinology and Metabolism. 2015;**100**(4):E572-E582

[98] Al-Hendy A, Diamond MP, Boyer TG, Halder SK. Vitamin D3 inhibits Wnt/β-catenin and mTOR signaling pathways in human uterine fibroid cells. The Journal of Clinical Endocrinology and Metabolism. 2016;**101**(4):1542-1551

[99] Corachán A, Ferrero H, Aguilar A, Garcia N, Monleon J, Faus A, et al. Inhibition of tumor cell proliferation in human uterine leiomyomas by vitamin D via Wnt/β-catenin pathway. Fertility and Sterility. 2019;**111**(2):397-407

[100] Reis FM, Bloise E, Ortiga-Carvalho TM. Hormones and pathogenesis of uterine fibroids. Best Practice & Research. Clinical Obstetrics & Gynaecology. 2016;**34**:13-24

[101] Borahay MA, Asoglu MR, Mas A, Adam S, Kilic GS, Al-Hendy A. Estrogen receptors and Signaling in fibroids: Role in pathobiology and therapeutic implications. Reproductive Sciences (Thousand Oaks, Calif.). 2017;**24**(9):1235-1244

[102] Moravek MB, Yin P, Ono M, Coon JS, Dyson MT, Navarro A, et al. Ovarian steroids, stem cells and uterine leiomyoma: Therapeutic implications. Human Reproduction Update. 2015;**21**(1):1-12

[103] Chegini N, Ma C, Tang XM, Williams RS. Effects of GnRH analogues, «add-back» steroid therapy, antiestrogen and antiprogestins on leiomyoma and myometrial smooth muscle cell growth and transforming growth factor-beta expression. Molecular Human Reproduction. 2002;**8**(12):1071-1078

[104] Hsieh YY, Chang CC, Tsai FJ, Tsai HD, Yeh LS, Lin CC, et al. Estrogen receptor thymine-adenine dinucleotide repeat polymorphism is associated with susceptibility to leiomyoma. Fertility and Sterility. 2003;**79**(1):96-99

[105] Al-Hendy A, Salama SA. Ethnic distribution of estrogen receptor-alpha polymorphism is associated with a higher prevalence of uterine leiomyomas in black Americans. Fertility and Sterility. 2006;**86**(3):686-693

[106] Ishikawa H, Reierstad S, Demura M, Rademaker AW, Kasai T, Inoue M, et al. High aromatase expression in uterine leiomyoma tissues of African-American women. The Journal of

Clinical Endocrinology and Metabolism. 2009;**94**(5):1752-1756

[107] Emrahi L, Behroozi J, Shahbazi S. Expression study of CYP19A1 gene in a cohort of Iranian leiomyoma patients. Egyptian Journal of Medical Human Genetics. 2018;**19**(3):197-200

[108] Al-Hendy A, Salama SA. Catechol-O-methyltransferase polymorphism is associated with increased uterine leiomyoma risk in different ethnic groups. Journal of the Society for Gynecologic Investigation. 2006;**13**(2):136-144

[109] Ishikawa H, Ishi K, Serna VA, Kakazu R, Bulun SE, Kurita T. Progesterone is essential for maintenance and growth of uterine leiomyoma. Endocrinology. 2010;**151**(6):2433-2442

[110] Kim JJ, Sefton EC. The role of progesterone signaling in the pathogenesis of uterine leiomyoma. Molecular and Cellular Endocrinology. 2012;**358**(2):223-231

Chapter 6

Elective Total Abdominal Hysterectomy for Symptomatic Uterine Fibroids: A Perspective on Its Impact on Women's Reproductive Health

Usman R. Yahaya, Eseoghene Dase, Shadrach M. Pius, Olakunle A. Azeez and Aliyu I. Lawan

Abstract

The chapter defines total abdominal hysterectomy (TAH), its historical background and epidemiology in the management of uterine fibroids in women who are in their reproductive years. The clinical presentations of uterine fibroids and circumstances in women of this age group that may indicate total abdominal hysterectomy as the option of surgical intervention is explained. The advantages of vaginal and laparoscopic approaches to hysterectomy were discussed. A detailed description of the surgical procedure is given with emphasis on its safety. Ways of avoiding intraoperative bleeding, during hysterectomy for uterine fibroids, were explained. The dilemma of decision making on the choice of the procedure by the gynaecologist and the patient is highlighted. Its impact, postoperatively, on the reproductive health of the women is discussed in perspective. Methods of fertility preservation in reproductive age women who are to undergo abdominal hysterectomy were mentioned. The chapter is concluded with a summary of its contents and the learning points.

Keywords: uterine fibroid, symptoms, abdominal hysterectomy, impact, reproductive health

1. Introduction

1.1 Uterine fibroid

1.1.1 Aetiology and epidemiology

Uterine fibroids are benign tumours of the smooth muscle of the uterus. Each fibroid arise from a single monoclonal cell of the smooth muscle of the myometrium. Their growth is affected by the female hormones, oestrogen and progesterone.

The exact aetiology of uterine fibroid is unknown. About 30% of fibroids have various chromosomal abnormalities ranging from trisomy, translocation and deletion. They are found commonly in women of reproductive age group. Other risk factors are being a black American, nulliparity, obesity, early menarche and family history of fibroids.

Fibroids are found in up to 80–90% of females worldwide. They are present in 20–25% of reproductive age women [1]. About one fifth of gynaecological clinic visits are as a result of fibroids and the estimated cost of their management is up to two billion dollars in the United State [1–3].

1.1.2 Symptoms and signs of uterine fibroids

Uterine fibroids are commonly asymptomatic, only about 30% of patients present with severe symptoms which varies in individual patient and according to the size and location of the fibroid in the uterus or degenerative changes within the fibroid. The commonest symptom is heavy menstrual bleeding. There may be pelvic pain in the form of dyspareunia, dysmenorrhea, and noncyclic pain. Abdominal protrusion and pressure of the mass on adjacent pelvic organs like the bladder and the rectum can result in urinary incontinence, urinary retention, hydro-nephrosis, constipation, and tenesmus respectively. Uterine fibroid is also associated with infertility and obstetric complications such as miscarriage, preterm labour/delivery, foetal malpresentation, and post-partum haemorrhage [4–6].

1.2 Hysterectomy

1.2.1 Definitions

Hysterectomy is the removal of the uterus. Total hysterectomy is the removal of both the body and the cervix of the uterus. Subtotal hysterectomy is the removal of the uterine corpus leaving the cervix in situ. Total abdominal hysterectomy is the removal of the uterus and the cervix through an abdominal incision. When the ovaries and fallopian tubes are removed in addition, it is referred to as total abdominal hysterectomy with salpingo-oophorectomy (TAH + BSO) or panhysterectomy [7].

1.2.2 Historical background

The first hysterectomy was a subtotal abdominal hysterectomy in which the uterus was removed and the cervix was left situ. It was performed by Charles Clay in 1843. It was Richardson who performed the first total abdominal hysterectomy in 1929. Over the years there had been modifications and improvements in the technique of the procedure. Total abdominal hysterectomy is preferred except in circumstances where it is difficult to perform with attendant increased risk of morbidity and mortality to the patient [8].

1.2.3 Surgical approach to hysterectomy

Hysterectomy can be performed through three different surgical approaches including; the abdominal, vaginal and laparoscopic route.

Laparoscopic approach has the advantages of shorter hospital stay, lower incidences of blood loss, postoperative pain, febrile morbidity and wound infections when compared with abdominal approach. The operating time is shorter in abdominal approach and the ability to navigate a distorted pelvic anatomy and perform extensive adhesiolysis safely is better than with laparoscopic hysterectomy. Vaginal approach has similar advantages as laparoscopic technique in terms of safety profiles with shorter operative time to its advantage. Several studies have shown that all outcomes are more favourable with vaginal hysterectomy compared with both laparoscopic and abdominal hysterectomy. Abdominal hysterectomy had been more common than the other routes until in recent times when laparoscopic methods are increasingly being preferred [9–11].

1.2.4 Indications for hysterectomy

Hysterectomy is a procedure that is indicated in both benign and malignant gynaecological conditions and some obstetric complications. Majority of the procedure are performed for benign conditions. The leading indications are, uterine fibroids, abnormal uterine bleeding, uterine prolapse, endometriosis and adenomyosis. Others are chronic pelvic pain, pelvic inflammatory disease, malignances of the uterus, cervix and ovary and postpartum haemorhage [12, 13].

1.2.5 Indications for total abdominal hysterectomy for the treatment of fibroids in women of reproductive age group

Removal of the uterus in women of reproductive age group comes with objectionable consequences. There is loss of fertility and menstrual flow. If the ovaries are removed in addition, premature menopause sets in. The indications for hysterectomy and the method in this age group should be well guided. In addition to vaginal hysterectomy as an alternative method of hysterectomy, the introduction of laparoscopic hysterectomy procedures had gained worldwide acceptance in recent times. In order to differentiate the areas of indication for each method, the German Society of Obstetrics and Gynecology (DGGG, Deutshe Gesellschaft fur Gynakologie and Geburtshiife) prepared a guideline; "Indications and methods of Hysterectomy for Benign Gynecology Disease". The following recommendations were made on the management of symptomatic uterine fibroids:

- It should first be verified that the symptoms are actually caused by the fibroids.
- Decision about treatment approach to be taken should be made together with the patient in consideration of her circumstances.
- Hysterectomy can be offered to those who do not wish for further childbirth, do not respond to alternative treatments or wish to undergo hysterectomy.
- The patients should be counselled about the success and failure rates of each method of fibroid treatment [14].

The surgical methods of approach to hysterectomy have been compared in several publications, including recommendation from the National Institute for health and Clinical Excellence (NICE) and the recommendation by the American College of Obstetricians and Gynecologists (ACOG). Vaginal hysterectomy was found to have the lowest complication rate and cost followed by laparoscopic hysterectomy procedures. It was recommended that abdominal hysterectomy should only be performed when there is a special indication for it (**Table 1**) [2, 14, 15].

- Large diffuse fibroids with uterine size greater than 18 weeks
- Anatomic distortion due to pelvic organ disease or adhesions
- Patient's choice after adequate counseling
- Lack of facilities and experience to offer patients alternative surgical methods

Table 1.
Indications for TAH as treatment for uterine fibroids in reproductive age women.

1.2.6 Abdominal hysterectomy rate in the management of uterine fibroids

Hysterectomy is the common gynaecological surgery performed in women worldwide. About 67% of hysterectomies in the UK were performed abdominally. Up to 39% of all hysterectomies performed annually in the United States were due to symptomatic uterine fibroids. In Germany, approximately 60% of hysterectomies, were done to treat uterine fibroids. In 2012, abdominal hysterectomy rates in the United States, Germany, Australia and Switzerland were reported to be 56%, 15%, 28.0% and 23.9% respectively [10, 13].

2. Hysterectomy in the reproductive age women; the dilemma of decision making

Hysterectomy is the definite treatment for uterine fibroids. However, it may not be an appropriate treatment option in reproductive age women due to loss of fertility and menstrual function; the hallmark of femininity. In addition to the loss of fecundity, it is also associated with low self-esteem, depression and anxiety [16, 17]. It may be a difficult decision for the women who wants to preserve their child bearing and or menstrual function.

On the other hand, hysterectomy is the only form of treatment that is associated with no recurrence. This benefit clearly outweighs the risk of recurrence, further investigations and treatments that are associated with uterine-preserving modalities. The cumulative rate of recurrence following myomectomy is 63–76% and majority of them will require further intervention [18]. Similarly, secondary hysterectomy was required for persistence of symptoms in 35% of patients after successful uterine artery embolization (UAE) for uterine fibroids [19]. Also, the re-intervention rate following fibroids treatment with MRI-guided high intensity ultrasound wave is 20.7%, this is largely due to symptomatic recurrence in 63.3% of cases [20]. Therefore, hysterectomy is an excellent option for reproductive age women who are not desirous of fertility and has completed their family size.

In addition, hysterectomy may be a life-saving procedure in the setting of uncontrollable haemorrhage during myomectomy. Besides, at 3-month after successful UAE, the risk of unintended hysterectomy is 1.5% [21]. In view of this, it is pertinent to counsel the women on the possibility of hysterectomy prior to these procedure and informed consent taken.

The choice of hysterectomy in women of reproductive age group depends on the severity of symptoms and the desire of the patient to mountain fertility. But, because there are uterine preserving alternative methods of treatment, decision making on the option of hysterectomy often puts both the patient and the gynaecologist in a state of dilemma. Often times, the patients have already decided on the treatment they want before coming for consultation. The gynaecologist is expected to provide them with information on the available options, their benefits and risks. They can then decide on the option that best suits them [2, 14].

3. Procedure of total abdominal hysterectomy

It is pertinent for the surgeon undertaking this procedure to bear in mind the risk of mortality and debilitating morbidity that are associated with it. However, there had been a rapid decline in morbidity and mortality over the years due to improvement in patient evaluation, refinement in surgical techniques and surgical duration. The surgeon needs to pay attention to these refinements to ensure a safe procedure. The technique of total abdominal hysterectomy in contemporary use is a modification of the classic Richardson method [8].

3.1 Preoperative preparations

Before the procedure it is necessary to take a brief history, a detailed physical and abdominal examination and to request biochemical and radiological tests as may be appropriate for the patient [22]. **Table 2** shows a list of such tests. The purpose of the evaluation is to;

- Delineate the size and extent of the uterine fibroid.
- Detect medical and other pelvic organs disease.
- Ascertain if the uterus is mobile or fixed.
- Choose the appropriate abdominal incision.
- Ascertain if the patient is fit for the procedure.

Investigation	Indication
• Full blood count (FBC)	To detect anaemia and evidence of infection
• Fasting blood sugar (FBS)	To screen for diabetes mellitus
• Electrolytes, urea & creatinine	To access renal function
• Pregnancy test (PT)	To rule out pregnancy
• Pap smear	To rule out cervical cancer
• Ultrasound scan of abdomen & pelvis	To access size of the uterus & detect other pelvic pathology
• Chest X-ray	To detect cardio-respiratory disease
• Intravenous pyelography (IVP)	To detect involvement of ureters and kidneys
• CT scan/MRI	To complement findings on USS if necessary

Table 2.
List of essential preoperative investigations.

The outcomes of evaluation are to be discussed with the patient. Medical co-morbidities detected especially anaemia, hypertension and diabetes mellitus should be treated appropriately prior to surgery. The patients should be counselled on the procedure plan and informed consent should be obtained. Bowel preparation may be necessary before the day of surgery to enhance exposure, reduce trauma to the bowel and prevent contamination of field during surgery. The pubic hair should be reduced with scissor or shaved with razor in the morning of surgery. A broad spectrum antibiotics like ceftaxidime or cefotaxime 2 g intravenously as prophylaxis against infection. Between 1 and 4 doses are given at 12 hourly intervals beginning 30 minutes before commencement of surgery.

Preventive measure against deep vein thrombosis and pulmonary embolism should be instituted in patients at risk. The use of sequential compression devices and low molecular weight heparin have been recommended [7, 8, 22–24].

3.1.1 Preoperative counselling

Abdominal hysterectomy may be accompanied by surgical morbidity and possibly mortality. Additionally, some patients do suffer from post-hysterectomy regret, especially among premenopausal women. Therefore, preoperative planning and decision-making should be comprehensive. The gynaecologist needs to build trust with the patient, the indications for the surgery and alternative treatment options have to be explained thoroughly to the patient. Potential for operative and postoperative complications should be discussed. Patient's desire for childbearing in the future and the possibilities should also be included in the counselling. Extensive pre-operative planning and execution of preventive measures have been associated with improved outcomes of surgery [25].

3.2 Operative technique

Patient is placed in supine position anaesthetized and an examination under anaesthesia is performed to unravel features that were not evident during initial physical examination and if there is need for specific preparation that have not been made. A Foley catheter is inserted into the bladder and the balloon is inflated with normal saline to retain it. The abdomen and vagina are cleaned with antiseptic solution and covered with sterile drapes with a window exposing the surgical site. For benign conditions like uterine fibroids, the abdomen is opened through a pfannenstiel incision on the skin. A midline subumbilical incision may be necessary when the uterine size is bigger than 12 weeks size or when there is a need for an increase in exposure. The peritoneal cavity is opened and explored for pathologies. The bowel is packed away from the pelvis by adjusting the surgical table to the Trendelenburg position and applying a large pack secured outside the abdomen with a clip on a long tape attached to it. The pack should be wet with normal saline before application to avoid damage to the bowel. A Balfour retractor is paced for exposure of the surgical fields. With the surgeon's hand in the pouch of Douglas, the uterus is lifted and elevated out of the pelvis (**Figure 1**). A large clamp is placed on each uterine cornu, such as to include the origins of the tubes and the round ligament to allow manipulation of the uterus. The right round ligament is stretched by manually deviating the uterus to the left side of the patient. It is clamped, cut and ligated around the midpoint. The same step is repeated on the left side of the patient. The anterior leaf of the broad ligament is then incised from this point to open the vesico-uterine folds of peritoneum.

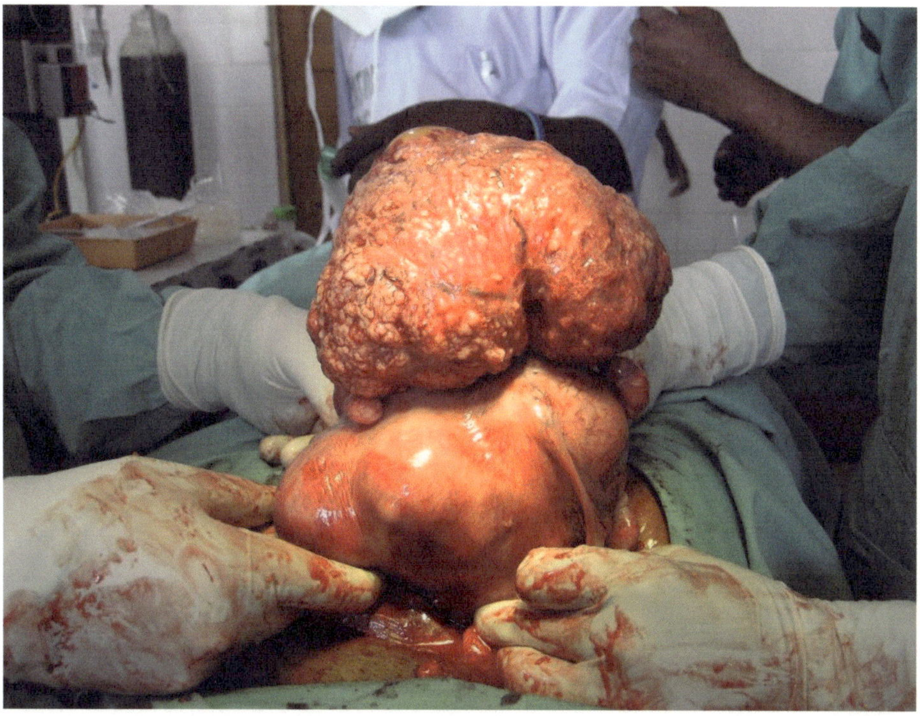

Figure 1.
Uterus riddled with fibroids lifted out of the pelvis through a midline sub-umbilical incision.

The bladder is dissected and reflected downward from the lower uterine segment, cervix and upper vaginal to lateralize the ureters and keep them out of harm's way. The incision is extended postero-laterally on the posterior leaf of the broad ligament, then directed superiorly, parallel and lateral to the infundibulopelvic ligament on the pelvic sidewall. The retroperitoneal space is thus opened by this manoeuvre. The soft areolar connective tissue is carefully separated with the index finger to expose the retroperitoneal structure.

The ureter is identified around the bifurcation of the common iliac artery and should be kept under direct vision. If the ovaries and the tubes are to be removed, they are moved together towards the uterus medially. A finger is used to create a window in the posterior leaf of the broad ligament and the infundibulopelvic ligament is double clamped cut and ligated. If the ovaries are to be retained, the tube is mobilise towards the uterus medially and the utero-ovarian ligament on each side is clamped, cut and ligated between the ovary and the free tube. Then the uterine artery is identified, the connective tissue overlying it is dissected. It is double clamped perpendicularly at the level of the internal os, cut and ligated. The same procedure is repeated on the other side. The rectum is mobilised from the posterior cervix by incising the posterior leaf of the broad ligament to the level of the utero-sacral ligament. The cardinal ligament and the utero-sacral ligaments are clamped, cut and ligated (**Figure 2**). The next step is to clamp the vaginal angles, open the anterior fornix with a scalpel and then expand the incision round the cervix. The edges of the vaginal are clamped at intervals, the vault is then closed antero-posteriorly. The cardinal and utero-sacral ligament stumps are sutured to the vaginal angle on both side to prevent postoperative vaginal vault prolapse and

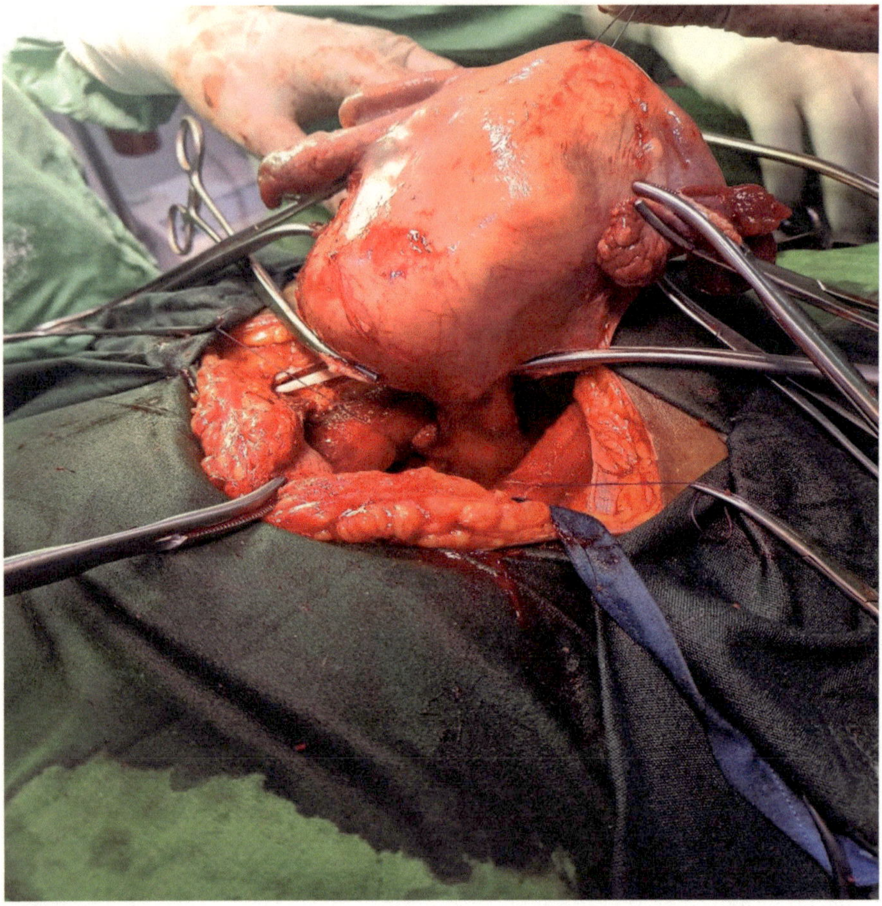

Figure 2.
Clamps on the upper stumps of the ligated and tied round ligaments, infundibulopelvic ligaments, uterine arteries and the cardinal ligaments.

enterocoele. The vault is covered by suturing the peritoneum of the anterior leaf of broad ligament to its posterior leaf with the stumps of the tubo-ovarian, cardinal and utero-sacral ligaments buried retroperitoneally. The bladder peritoneum is suture, to the pouch of Douglas. The pelvis is inspected to ensure that the stumps are not bleeding (**Figure 3**). The peritoneum is lavaged with normal saline. The anterior abdominal wall incision is then closed in layers with subcuticular suture to the skin [7, 8, 23, 24, 26, 27].

The hysterectomy specimen is sent to histopathology laboratory for report (**Figure 4**).

3.2.1 Modification of technique due to uterine fibroid

Modifications to the operative technique may be necessary if the pelvic anatomy is distorted due to; large uterus, broad ligament fibroid and cervical fibroid. In these circumstances, there may be limited space in the pelvis and access may be difficult. The ureters are displaced laterally and the blood vessels are usually dilated and tortuous. There is a high risk of injury to ureters, uterus and bladder. The risks associated

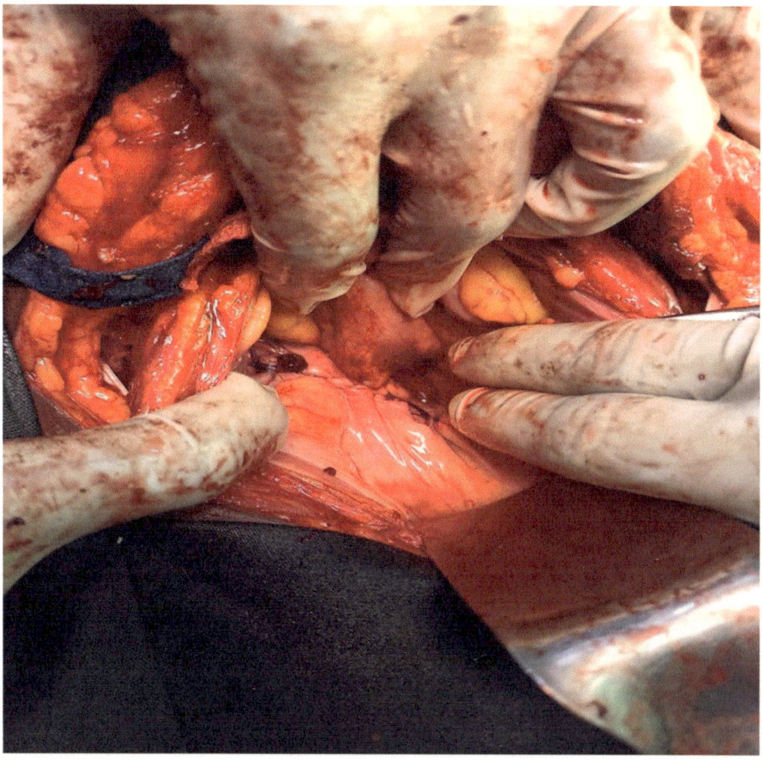

Figure 3.
Reperitonization of the pelvis with all the stumps buried retroperitonially.

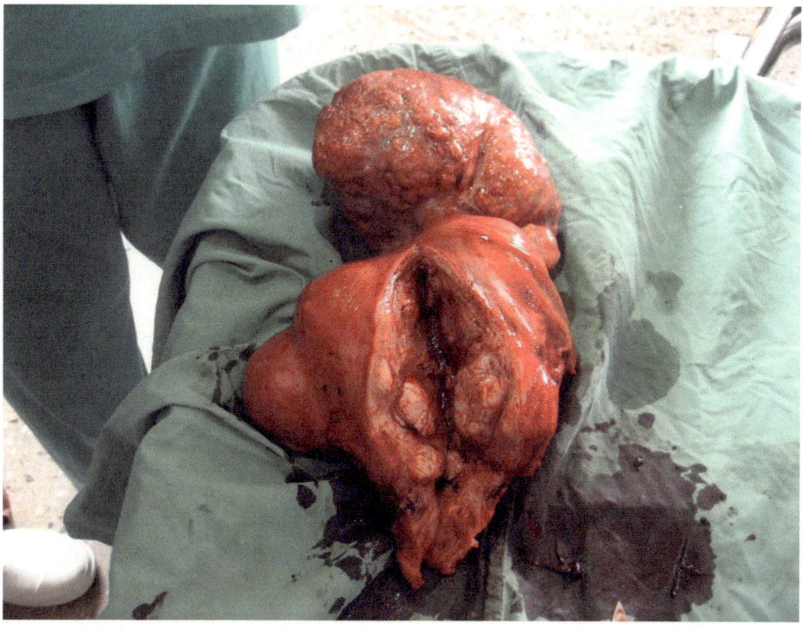

Figure 4.
Hysterectomy specimen sent for histopathology report.

with these situations are preventable. The uterus needs to be correctly oriented by locating landmark anatomical structures like the round ligaments, fallopian tubes and the ovaries. The procedure should start from the pelvic side wall that is most easily accessible. Adequate exposure and access to pelvic sidewall can be achieved with a debulking myomectomy. The largest most accessible fibroid should be removed first in a rapid manner to control haemorrhage [8, 26, 27].

3.3 Histopathology of uterine fibroids

Uterine fibroids are also called leiomyoma derived from leio, meaning smooth, myo – muscle and –oma is a suffix indicating a benign neoplasm. They are also referred to as fibromyomas. They are benign mesenchymal neoplasm arising from smooth muscle tissue of the myometrium of the uterus. However, there could arise from the cervix and broad ligament [2].

Grossly, they appear firm, greyish white to tan nodules of varying sizes ranging from grain size in millimetres to over 25 cm in widest diameter. Sizes as large as 50–60 cm had been reported [28, 29]. It could be single but most commonly, they are multiple. They have greyish white whorled appearance on cut surfaces.

Following hysterectomy specimen, there could be complete or partial distortion of the uterine architecture. They could be pedunculated and extend from the serosal surface of the uterus. On cut section, they appear as well circumscribed nodular masses below the endometrial lining (submucous), within the myometrium (intramural) or below the serosa (subserosal). In some cases, the submucous fibroids could be pedunculated, bulge and dilate the endometrial cavity. The pedunculated masses could protrude down to the cervix. Most that protrude through the cervix might have an ulcerated surface with areas of necrosis and haemorrhage (**Figures** 5 and **6**).

Various degenerative changes impact on the appearance. There could be cysts within the mass containing clear myxoid to clear fluid in cystic degeneration. In red degeneration, they appear red to brown on cut surfaces. In calcific degeneration, the tissue could be hard with chalky white appearance on cut surfaces with gritty sensation. A nodule could be transformed into a 'stone' due to extensive calcification. In hyaline degeneration, they could be yellowish in areas [30].

Microscopically, they are composed of proliferating smooth muscle cells which are spindle shaped disposed in interlacing and anastomosing fascicles and bundles. The nuclei are elongated with blunt ends and inconspicuous nucleoli. The cytoplasm is moderate, eosinophilic and indistinct. Mitotic figures are infrequent, less than 5 per 10 high power field.

The neoplasm is fairly circumscribed and exerts pressure on the surrounding normal myometrium with formation of a pseudocapsule [29]. The intervening stroma can be extensively hyalinised in hyaline change. Myxoid stroma change could also be seen. There may be areas of dystrophic calcification. In cystic degeneration, the cyst is devoid of epithelial lining. In large leiomyoma, there can be areas of necrosis. Areas of haemorrhage and congested vascular channels can be seen.

Special names are being given to particular features. A cellular leiomyoma is given when there is hyper-cellularity than normal [31]. This is usually more cellular than the surrounding normal myometrium. The component cells could resemble epithelial cells and are thus called epithelioid leiomyoma. A mitotically active leiomyoma is seen when the mitotic count is above 5. The count is about 6–20/10 high power field.

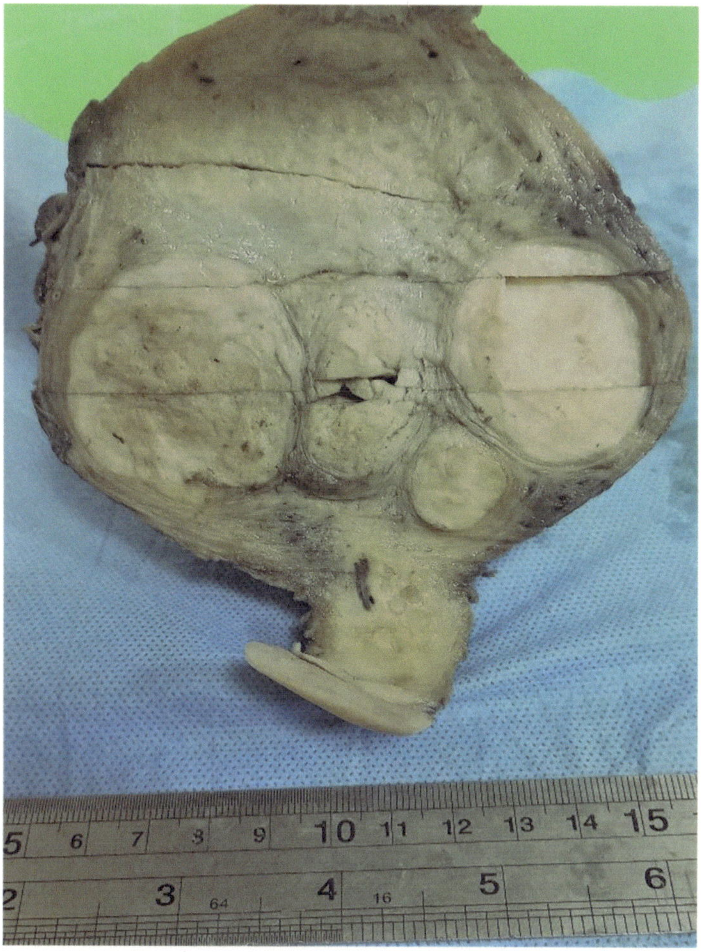

Figure 5.
A enlarged hysterectomy specimen with distorted architecture with multiple intramural fibroid nodules.

However, these mitotic figures are normal. A bizzare or symplastic or atypical leiomyoma is when the cells show cytonuclear pleomorphism with large atypical nuclei. Giant cells could be seen. However, there is no increase mitotic count or necrosis. This is important to differentiate from leiomyosarcoma which is the malignant counterpart where there is increased cellularity, pleomorphism, increased mitosis and necrosis (**Figures** 7 and **8**).

Leiomyoma express oestrogen and progesterone receptors. They are positive for desmin, smooth muscle actin, muscle specific actin and caldesmon. They are positive for vimentin. Epithelial membrane antigen is usually negative. However, occasional positivity for cytokeratin does occur [31, 32].

3.4 Postoperative care

The care given to patients post abdominal hysterectomy is about the same for any other major abdominal surgery. A Summary is presented in **Table 3** [7, 8, 24].

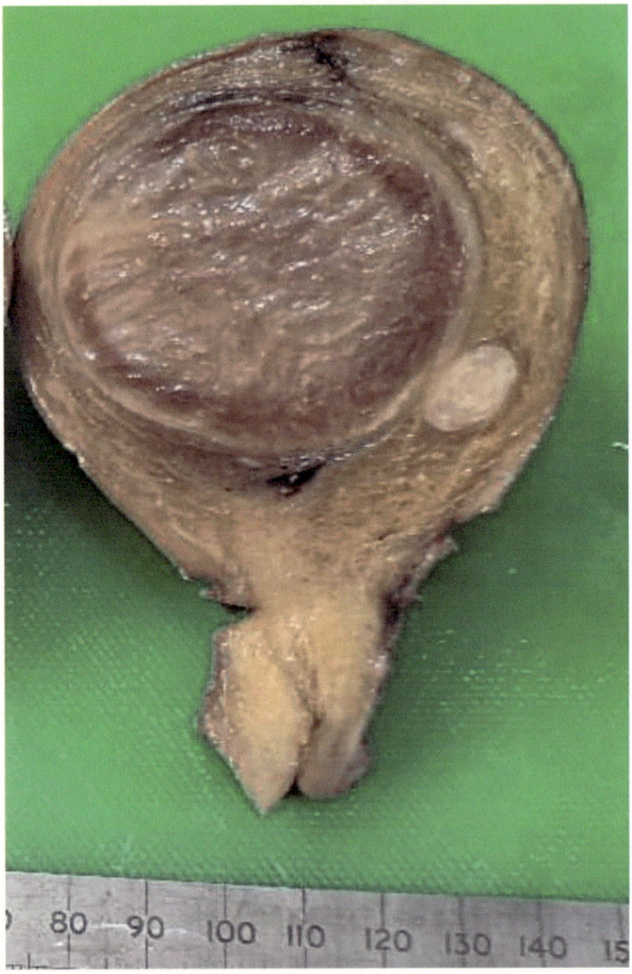

Figure 6.
A hysterectomy specimen with a large degenerate submucous fibroid compressing the endometrial cavity. Another small intramural fibroid is noted.

3.5 Complications of abdominal hysterectomy

Abdominal hysterectomy is associated with the risks of morbidity and mortality. Complication can occur intraoperatively, postoperatively, or both. They can be immediate or long term. The major complications are listed in **Table 4**.

Obesity, diabetes mellitus, large uterus, cervical fibroids, adhesion and improper surgical technique have been identified as risk factors to complications.

Serious complications are comparatively rare. Various complication rates have been reported ranging between 1.4% and 4.4%. Infection complications after abdominal hysterectomy are most common with the rate ranging from 2.5% to 10.5%. Genito-urinary tract injury is estimated to occur at a rate of 1.2%, with 75% of it occurring intraoperatively. Haemorrhage requiring blood transfusion is reported from different studies at a rate of 1–6%. The rate of blood transfusion is 4–6%. Deep vein thrombosis, bowel injury, vaginal vault, prolapse, neuropathy and death are all relatively less common with a rate less than 1% [8, 24, 33–35].

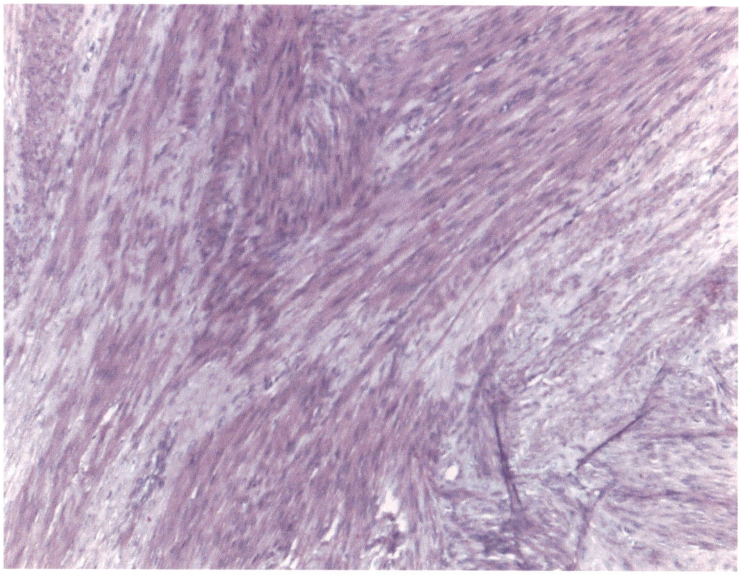

Figure 7.
H&Ex400—histologic section showing proliferating spindle cells disposed in interlacing fascicles.

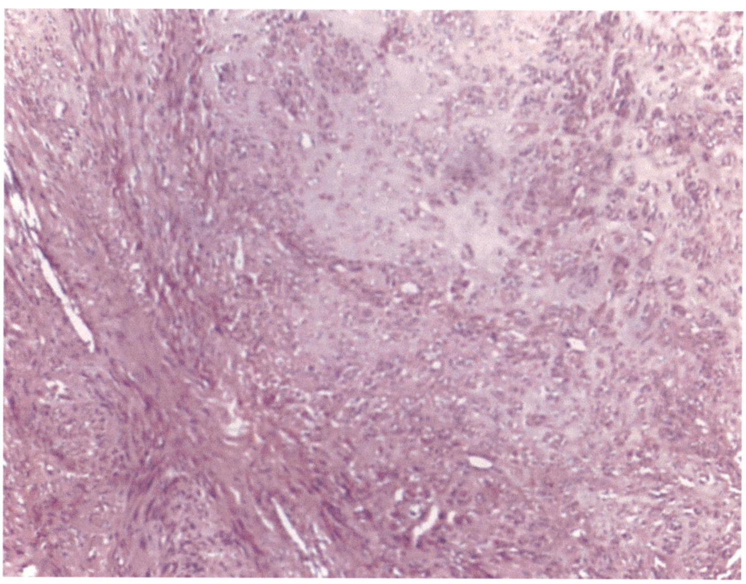

Figure 8.
H&Ex400—histologic section showing focal stromal hyalinization.

3.5.1 Avoidance of intraoperative bleeding during abdominal hysterectomy for uterine fibroid

Therefore, minimising the amount of intraoperative bleeding is essential to reducing associated preoperative morbidity and mortality. Under normal circumstances, adequate attention to proper surgical technique is enough to secure haemostosis during abdominal hysterectomy. However, additional preventive and

• Administration of intravenous fluids for the first 24 h especially if patient is feeling nauseated or vomiting.
• Indwelling Foley catheter should be discontinued the morning after surgery if there is no bladder or ureteric injury.
• Pain relief with appropriate analgesia
• Encourage ambulation as early as the afternoon or evening on the day of surgery.
• Commencement of oral intake within 24 h after surgery
• Removal of skin sutures on the seventh post operative day.
• Discharge patient after removal of skin sutures if there are no complications.
• Patient to avoid vaginal intercourse for up to 6 weeks.
• Patient to report any symptoms and signs of complications such as fever, pain, vomiting, purulent discharge per vagina or from the wound and severe bleeding per vagina.

Table 3.
Postoperative care and instructions on discharge.

Complications
Immediate
• Post operative pyrexia
• Severe haemorrhage
• Bladder, ureteral and bowel injury
• Surgical site infection
• Anaesthetic complications
• Deep vein thrombosis
• Neuropathy
Long term
• Vagina vault prolapse
• Pelvic adhesion
• Urinary incontinence
• Premature menopause
• Regret

Table 4.
Complications of abdominal hysterectomy.

therapeutic measures may be necessary in the presence of risk factors for bleeding. Techniques that have been used to prevent or control heavy bleeding during abdominal hysterectomy include; prophylactic vasopressin, preoperative misoprostol, ligaSure, ligation of uterine and iliac arteries, and trans arterial embolization of uterine or internal iliac arteries using interventional radiologic procedures. These procedures can be performed both prior to hysterectomy and for persistent bleeding after hysterectomy. Dilute vasopressin solution injected about 1 cm media to the uterine arteries has been found to reduce blood loss by 40%. Studies have shown ligaSure vessel-sealing device to be more effective in securing haemostasis than misoprostol and tranexamic acid.

Blood loss is effectively reduced through bilateral uterine artery ligation. The ascending branches of the uterine arteries are ligated with a suture at the level of the vesicouterine peritoneal reflection. The suture is passed lateral to the vessels through an avascular area of the blood ligament close to the cervix. Ligation or stapling off the internal iliac artery significantly reduces blood loss. After insulating the artery, ligation is done about 2 cm distal to the origin of the posterior branch to limit collateral flow to the uterus and prevent gluteal ischemia [36–38].

3.5.2 Therapeutic mappings of uterine fibroids during labour

Uterine fibroids have been found in about 3–12% of pregnant women and are also associated with adverse pregnancy outcomes. There is increased risk of peripartum haemorrhage and caesarean section due to fetal malpresentation. Postpartum haemorhage is one of the leading courses of maternal mortality [35, 39, 40].

For a pregnant woman in labour with coexisting uterine fibroids, adequate preparations should be made for the treatment of potential complications due to the fibroids. In case of obstructed labour, the therapeutic options are; caesarean section with myomectomy and or caesarean hysterectomy as may be indicated [41].

Interventions that may be necessary for persistent severe postpartum haemorrhage include, selective uterine artery embolization or ligation, ligation of the internal iliac artery and postpartum hysterectomy. There should be no delay in carrying out any of these interventions as may be necessary [37, 38].

4. Impact of TAH on reproductive health of women of reproductive age group

Total abdominal hysterectomy for uterine fibroids has huge impacts on women's sexual and reproductive health. These impacts could be positive or negative.

Positive impacts of TAH include symptomatic relief from symptoms of fibroids, improved sexual functions and improved quality of life [42]. Being a definitive treatment for uterine fibroids, TAH provides permanent relief from symptoms such as menorrhagia, dysmenorrhoea and pressure symptoms. Getting relief from these distressing symptoms improves their quality of life by reduced hospital visits due to anaemia and dysmenorrhea.

Also, majority of patients are reported to have improved sexual function after TAH [43–45]. This improvement in sexual function is probably due to improved overall health due to higher haemoglobin levels, and relief from pelvic pressure and pain. The permanent amenorrhoea also results in less impediment to regular sexual intercourse.

Since TAH involves total removal of the cervix and uterine corpus, a remote positive impact is the elimination of both cervical and endometrial cancer risk, and upper genital tract infections. This eliminates the need for regular pap smears and treatment for both premalignant cervical lesions and pelvic inflammatory disease. Reduced incidence of depressive illness has been reported among patients who had hysterectomy for uterine fibroids and this improvement in mental health is likely due to relief from the debilitating effect of menorrhagia, dysmenorrhea and abdominal distension from huge fibroids [46]. The complete sense of cure from TAH is also likely to contribute to the improvements in the mood of these patients.

Negative impacts of TAH include psychological problems and sexual difficulties. One major psychological challenge some women face after hysterectomy is the loss of sense of femininity which could result in low self-esteem and impaired sexual function [47, 48]. Also, TAH in younger and nulliparous women result in loss of reproductive capacity with a consequent adverse psychologic effect on the woman and her partner [44]. These patients may also experience worsening of anxiety disorders.

In addition, when bilateral salpingo-oophorectomy (BSO) is performed together with TAH in reproductive age women, there is significant decline in sexual function and increased psychosocial health risk [49]. Some studies have suggested reduced sexual satisfaction due to removal of the cervix in TAH; however, the evidence is inconclusive. Other studies have found no significant difference in sexual function in women who underwent TAH compared to those who had sub-total hysterectomy.

While many patients will have positive experiences following TAH for symptomatic uterine fibroids, others will have less desirable experiences. Adequate preoperative counselling will enable patients with uterine fibroids to measure their expectations and adjust appropriately.

4.1 Methods of fertility preservation in premenopausal women undergoing abdominal hysterectomy

For reproductive-age women with uterine fibroids desiring future childbearing, the best option is to avoid hysterectomy. Alternative treatment methods that preserve the uterus and fertility such as myomectomy, and uterine artery embolization (UAE), high intensity focused ultrasound (HIFU) and medical therapy should be adopted where possible [50, 51].

However, hope is not lost for those women in whom hysterectomy is inevitable. Assisted Reproductive Technologies (ART) have provided an array of options for fertility preservation to help them have their own genetic children. These include; controlled ovarian stimulation and cryopreservation of oocytes or embryos and cryopreservation of ovarian tissue. There is also the option of third-party reproduction which includes donated oocytes or embryos and surrogacy [52].

4.1.1 Embryos and oocytes cryopreservation, ovarian tissue cryopreservation and surrogacy

A woman who has been scheduled to undergo hysterectomy is given ovulation induction drugs to stimulate production of excess oocytes. These are either cryopreserved or used to produce embryos, through in vitro fertilisation techniques, for cryopreservation. If the time to surgery does not permit this process, her ovarian tissue can be cryopreserved or donor oocytes and embryos can be used. For the process of fertility to complete, the woman will need the help of a surrogate mother to serve as gestational carrier after hysterectomy. It is to be noted that embryo cryopreservation, donor embryo, and surrogacy have generated a lot of ethical, moral, and legal issues. The patient should be referred to specialised fertility center for proper counselling and treatment [53–55].

5. Conclusion

In conclusion, uterine fibroids are benign tumours of the smooth muscle of the uterus. They are present in 20–25% of reproductive age women. Hysterectomy is the definitive treatment and there are 3 different methods of approach to it, abdominal hysterectomy, vaginal hysterectomy and laparoscopic hysterectomy procedures. Between 30 and 60% of hysterectomies are performed to treat uterine fibroids and about 15–59% are reported to be abdominal hysterectomy.

Total abdominal hysterectomy is the removal of the uterus and the cervix through an abdominal incision. If the ovaries and the tubes are removed in addition, it is referred to as total abdominal hysterectomy with bilateral salpingo-oophorectomy. The procedure is relatively safe with low morbidity and mortality rates. It has both positive and negative impacts on the reproductive health of women. The major consequences in reproductive age women are loss of fertility and premature menopause. The choice of hysterectomy in this age group depends on the severity of the symptoms and the desire of the patients to maintain fertility. There are alternatives modes of treating uterine fibroids which are uterus-preserving. There are also methods of fertility preservation for those in whom hysterectomy is unavoidable. Therefore, the gynaecologist is expected to counsel the patients adequately on these so that they can decide on the option that best suits them and their decision should be respected.

Acknowledgements

The authors thank Mr. Olagunju Femi D for Typing and arrangement.

Conflict of interest

The authors declare no conflict of interest.

Acronyms and abbreviations

ACOG	American College of Obstetricians and Gynecologists
ART	Assisted Reproductive Technology
BSO	bilateral salpingo-oophorectomy
DGGG	Deutshe Gesellschaft fur Gynakologie and Geburtshiife
GSOG	German Society of Obstetrics and Gynecology
FBC	full blood count
FBS	fasting blood sugar
HIFU	high intensity focused ultrasound
IVP	intravenous pyelography
NICE	National Institute for Health and Clinical Excellence
PT	pregnancy test
TAH	total abdominal hysterectomy
UAE	uterine artery embolization

Author details

Usman R. Yahaya[1*], Eseoghene Dase[2], Shadrach M. Pius[3], Olakunle A. Azeez[4] and Aliyu I. Lawan[5]

1 Department of Obstetrics and Gynaecology, Modibbo Adama University Teaching Hospital, Yola, Nigeria

2 Department of Obstetrics and Gynaecology, Cedarcrest Hospitals, Abuja, Nigeria

3 Department of Obstetrics and Gynaecology, Maitama District Hospital, Abuja, Nigeria

4 Department of Obstetrics and Gynaecology, Federal Teaching Hospital, Gombe, Nigeria

5 Department of Histopathology, Federal Teaching Hospital, Gombe, Nigeria

*Address all correspondence to: uryahaya@yahoo.com

References

[1] Hammer A, Rositch AF, Kathleen J. Global epidemiology of hysterectomy: Possible impact on gynaecology cancer rate. AMJ Obstetrics and Gynaecology. 2015;**213**(1):23-29

[2] De La Cruiz M, Buchanan EM. Uterine fibroids: Diagnosis and treatment. American Family Physician. 2017;**95**(2):100-107

[3] Yang Q, Ciebiera M, Bariani MV, Ali M, Elkafas H, Boyer TG, et al. Comprehensive review of uterine fibroids: Developmental origin, pathogenesis and treatment. Endocrinology Review. 2022;**43**(4):678-719. DOI: 10.1210/endrev/bnab039

[4] Duke CMP, Cholokian D, Sheib SA. Uterine leiomyomas. In: Johnson CT, Hallock JL, Bienstok JL, Fox HE, Wallach EE, editors. The Johns Hopkins Manual of Gynaecology and Obstetrics. 5th ed. Philadelphia: Wolters Kluwer; 2015. pp. 496-503

[5] Giuliani E, As-Sanie S, Marsh E. Epidemiology and management of uterine fibroids. International Journal of Gynecology & Obstetrics. 2020;**149**(1):3-9. DOI: 10.1002/ijgo.13102

[6] Ahmad A, Kumar M, Bhoi NR, Badruddeen A, Khan MI, et al. Diagnosis and management of uterine fibroids: Current trends and future strategies. Journal of Basic and Clinical Physiology and Pharmacology. 2023;**34**(3):291-310. DOI: 10.1515/jbcpp-2022-0219

[7] Saxena R. Tips and Tricks in Operative Obstetrics and Gynaecology. New Delhi: Jaypee Brothers Medical Publishers; 2011. pp. 440-457

[8] Swaim LS. Abdominal hysterectomy. In: Handa VL, Vanle L, editors. Te Linde's Operative Gynaecology. 12th ed. Philadelphia: Lippincott Williams & Wilkins; 2020. pp. 365-387

[9] Aarts JW, Nieboer TE, Johnson N, Tavender E, Garry R, Mol BWJ, et al. Surgical approach to hysterectomy for benign gynaecological disease. Cochrane Database of Systematic Reviews. 2015;**2015**:CD003677. DOI: 10.1002/14651858.CD003677

[10] Lycke KD, Kahlert J, Damgaard R, Mogensen O, Hammer A. Trends in hysterectomy incidence rates during 2000-2015 in Denmark: Shifting from abdominal to minimally invasive surgical procedures. Clinical Epidemiology. 2021;**13**:407-416. DOI: 10.2147/CLEP.S300394

[11] Dedden SJ, Geomini PM, Huirne JA, Bongers MY. Vaginal and laparoscopic hysterectomy as an outpatient procedure: A systematic review. European Journal of Obstetrics & Gynecology and Reproductive Biol. 2017;**216**:212-223

[12] Sakko Y, Aimqambetova G, Terzic M, Ukybassova T, Bapayeva G, Gusmanov A, et al. The prevalence, indications, outcomes of the Most common major gynaecological surgeries in Kazakhstan and recommendations for potential improvements into public health and clinical practice: Analysis of the National Electronic Healthcare System (2014-2019). International Journal of Environmental Research and Public Health. 2022;**19**(22):14679. DOI: 10.3390/ijerph192214679

[13] Alqahtani NH, Albayat MI, Al Nashwan YA, Alnemer AM. Pathologic profile of hysterectomy cases in Saudi Arabia: A Tertiary Center Experience. Saudi Journal of Medicine & Medical

Sciences. 2023;**11**(3):257-263. DOI: 10.4103/sjmms.sjmms43822

[14] Neis KJ, Zubke W, Fehr M, Romer T, Tamussino K, Nothacker M. Hysterectomy for benign disease. Deutsches Arztebl International. 2016;**113**(14):242-249. DOI: 10.3238/arztebl.2016.0242

[15] ACOG committee Opinion No. 444. Choosing the route of hysterectomy for benign disease. Obstetrics and Gynecology. 2009;**114**:1156-1158

[16] Bukar M, Audu BM, Yahaya UR. Hysterectomy for benign gynaecological conditions at Gombe, north eastern Nigeria. Nigerian Medical Journal. 2010;**51**:35-38

[17] Laughlin-Tommaso SK, Khan Z, Smith CY, Rocca WA, Stewart EA. Long-term risk of de novo mental health conditions after hysterectomy with ovarian conservation: A cohort study. Menopause. 2020;**27**(1):33-42

[18] Kotani Y, Tobiume T, Fujishima R, Shigeta M, Takaya H, Nakai H, et al. Recurrence of uterine myoma after myomectomy: Open versus laparoscopic myomectomy. The Journal of Obstetrics and Gynaecology Research. 2018;**44**(2):298-302

[19] de Bruijn AM, Ankum WM, Reekers JA, Birnie E, van der Kooij SM, Volkers NA, et al. Uterine artery embolization vs hysterectomy in the treatment of symptomatic uterine fibroids. 10-year outcomes from the randomized EMMY trial. American Journal of Obstetrics and Gynaecology. 2016;**215**(6):745.e1-745.e12

[20] Li W, Jiang Z, Deng X, Xu D. Long-term follow-up outcome and reintervention analysis of ultrasound-guided high intensity focused ultrasound treatment for uterine fibroids. International Journal of Hyperthermia. 2020;**37**(1):1046-1051

[21] Pron G, Mocarski CM, Colgan T, Bennet J, Common A, et al. Hysterectomy for complications after uterine embolization for leiomyoma: Results of a Canadian multicenter clinical trial. Journal of American Association Gynaecology Laparoscope. 2003;**10**(1):99-106

[22] Hepner DL. The role of testing in the preoperative evaluation. Cleveland Clinic Journal of Medicine. 2009;**76**(4):522-527

[23] Bristow RE. Total abdominal hysterectomy. In: Cundiff GW, Azziz R, Briston RE, editors. Te Linde's Atlas of Gynaecologic Surgery. Philadelphia: Lippincott Williams & Wilkins; 2014. pp. 15-24

[24] Munshi A, Munshi S. Abdominal hysterectomy. In: Puri R, Malhotra N, editors. Operative Obstetrics and Gynaecology. New Delhi: Jaypee Brothers Medical Publishers; 2009. pp. 486-493

[25] Björkström LM, Wodlin NB, Nilsson L, Kjølhede P. The impact of preoperative assessment and planning on the outcome of benign hysterectomy – A systematic review. Geburtshilfe und Frauenheilkunde. 2021;*81*(2):200-213. DOI: 10.1055la-1263-0811

[26] Lopes T, Spirtos NM, Hilton P, Monaghan JM, editors. Bonney's Gynecological Surgery. 12th ed. Hoboken, New Jersey, USA: John Wiley; 2018. pp. 107-116

[27] Hiramatsu Y. Hysterectomy for cervical and intraligamental fibroids. Surgical Journal (NY). 2020;**6**(1):s2-s10. DOI: 10.1055/5-0039-1698419

[28] Viva W, Juhi D, Kristin A, et al. Massive uterine fibroid: A diagnostic dilemma: A case report and review of the literature. Journal of Medical Case Reports. 2021;**15**:344. DOI: 10.1186/s13256-021-02959-3

[29] Tanos V, Berry KE. Benign and malignant pathology of the uterus. Best Practice & Research Clinical Obstetrics & Gynaecology. 2018;**46**:12-30

[30] Naz S, Rehman A, Riyaz A, Jehangir F, Naeem S, Iqbal T. Leiomyoma: Its variants and secondary changes A five-year study. Journal of Ayub Medical College Abbottabad. 2019;**31**(2):192-195

[31] Griffin BB, Feng Y, Saini P, Lu X, Bulun S, Chakravarti D, et al. Histological and molecular analysis of cellular leiomyoma with sclerosis: Linked to HMGA 2 overexpression. Histopathology. 2022;**81**(5):587-599. DOI: 10.1111/his.14732

[32] Porter AE, Kho KA, Gwin K. Mass lesions of the myometrium: Interpretation and management of unexpected pathology. Current Opinion in Obstetrics & Gynaecology. 2019;**31**(5):349-355. DOI: 10.1097/GCO.0000000000000569

[33] Metter L, Schollmeyer T, Tinelli A, Malvasi A, Alkatout I. Complications of uterine fibroids and their management, surgical management of fibroids, laparoscopy and hysterectomy, versus hysterectomy, hemorrhage adhesions and complications. Obstetrics and Gynaecology International. 2012;**2012**:8. DOI: 10.1155/2012/79/248

[34] Pearson C, Haniel L, Geller EJ. Complication of hysterectomy. Obstetrics and Gynaecology. 2013;**121**(3):654-673. DOI: 10.1097/AOG.obo 13e3182841594

[35] Ramdhan RC, Loukas M, Tubbs RS. Anatomical complications of hysterectomy: A review. Clinical Anatomy. 2017;**30**(7):946-952. DOI: 10.1002/ca.22962

[36] Hafidh B, Latifah HM, Gari A, Alshahrani MS, AlSghan R, Alkhamis WH, et al. Vasopressin to control blood loss during hysterectomy: A systematic review0 and meta-analysis of randomized controlled trials. Journal of Minimally Invasive Gynecol. 2022;**29**(3):355-364.e2. DOI: 10.1016/j.jmig.2021.10.003

[37] Gingold JA, Chichura A, Harnegie MP, Kho RM. Perioperative interventions to minimize blood loss at the time of hysterectomy for uterine leiomyomas: A systematic review and meta-analysis. Journal of Minimally Invasive Gynaecology. 2019;**26**(7):123455-121252. DOI: 10.1016/j.jmig.2019.04.021

[38] Choubey V, Werner EF. Complications of labour and delivery. In: Johnson CT, Hallock JL, Bienstock JL, Fox HE, Wallack EE, editors. The Johns Hopkins Manual of Gynecology and Obstetrics. 5th ed. Philadelphia: Wolters Kluwer; 2015. pp. 104-115

[39] Parazzini F, Tozzi L, Bianchi S. Pregnancy outcome and uterine fibroids. Best Practice & Research Clinical Obstetrics & Gynaecology. 2016;**34**:74-84. DOI: 10.1016/j.bpobgyn.2015.11.017

[40] Karlsen K, Kesmodel US, Mogensen O, Humaidan P, Ravn P. Relationship between a uterine fibroid diagnosis and the risk of adverse obstetrical outcomes: A cohort study. BMJ Open. 2020;**10**(2):e032104. DOI: 10.1136/bmjopen-2019-032104

[41] An J, Lin J, Sun P. Myomectomy for a large submucosal fibroid at the

time of caesarean section. Journal of College Physicians and Surgical Pakistan. 2022;**32**(3):383-385. DOI: 10.29271/jcpsp.2022.03,383

[42] Lonnée-Hoffmann R, Pinas I. Effects of hysterectomy on sexual function. Current Sex Health Reports. 2014;**6**(4):244-251

[43] Dedden SJ, Werner MA, Steinweg J, Lissenberg-Witte BI, Huirne JAF, Geomini PMAJ, et al. Hysterectomy and sexual function: A systematic review and meta-analysis. The Journal of Sexual Medicine. 2023;**20**(4):447-466

[44] Solbrække KN, Bondevik H. Absent organs – present selves: Exploring embodiment and gender identity in young Norwegian women's accounts of hysterectomy. International Journal of Quality Studies in Health Well-being. 2015;**10**:26720. DOI: 10.3402/qhw.v10.26720. PMID: 25937002; PMCID: PMC4417683

[45] Fram KM, Saleh SS, Sumrein IA. Sexuality after hysterectomy at University of Jordan Hospital: A teaching hospital experience. Archives of Gynecology and Obstetrics. 2013;**287**(4):703-708

[46] Okunlola MA, Umuerri C, Omigbodun OO, Morhason-Bello IO, Okonkwo SN, Ojengbede OA. Pattern of mental ill health morbidities following hysterectomy for benign gynaecological disorders among Nigerian women. International Journal of Mental Health System. 2009;**3**:1-5

[47] Danesh M, Hamzehgardeshi Z, Moosazadeh M, Shabani-Asrami F. The effect of hysterectomy on women's sexual function: A narrative review. Medical Archieve (Sarajevo, Bosnia Herzegovina). 2015;**69**(6):387-392

[48] Afiyah RK, Wahyuni CU, Prasetyo B, Winarno DD. Recovery time period and quality of life after hysterectomy. Journal of Public Health Research. 2020;**9**(2):176-178

[49] Radosa JC, Meyberg-Solomayer G, Kastl C, Radosa CG, Mavrova R, Gräber S, et al. Influences of different hysterectomy techniques on patients' postoperative sexual function and quality of life. The Journal of Sexual Medicine. 2014;**11**(9):2342-2350

[50] Napoli A, Alfieri G, Andrani F, Scipione R, Manganaro L, Pecorini F, et al. Uterine myomas: Focused ultrasound surgery. Seminars in Ultrasound, CT and MRI. 2021;**42**(1):25-36. DOI: 10.1053//sult.2020.08.001

[51] Daniels J, Middleton LJ, Cheed V, McKinnon W, Rana D, Sirkeci F, et al. Uterine artery embolisation versus myomectomy for premenopausal women with uterine fibroids wishing to avoid hysterectomy: The FEMME RCT. Health Technology Assess. 2022;**26**(22):1-74. DOI: 3310/ZDEG 6110

[52] Oktay K, Harvey BE, Partridge AH, Quinn GP, Reinecke J, Taylor HS, et al. Fertility preservation in patients with cancer: ASCO clinical practice guideline update. Journal of Clinical Oncol. 2018;**36**(19):1994-2001. DOI: 10.1200/JCO.2018.78.1914

[53] Rienzi L, Gracia C, Maggiulli R, LaBarbera AR, Kaser DJ, Ubalai FM, et al. Oocyte, embryo and blastocyst cryopreservation in ART. Systematic review and meta-analysis comparing slow-freezing versus vitrification to produce evidence for the development of global guidance. HUM Report Update. 2017;**23**:139155. DOI: 10.1093/humupd/dmw038

[54] van Oosbree A, Von Wald T. Gestational surrogacy and ethical considerations. SD Medicine. 2023;**76**(2):*72-75*

[55] Donnez J, Dolmans MM. Fertility preservation in men and women: Where are we in 2021? Are we rising to the challenge? Fertility and Sterility. 2021;**115**(5):1089-1090. DOI: 10.1016/j.fertnstert.2021. 03.028

Chapter 7

A Systematic Review on Uterine Leiomyoma: From Pathogenomics to Therapeutics

Sonia Narwal, Minakshi Vashist, Rohit Kaushik, Vandana Kalra, Reetu Hooda and Sunita Singh

Abstract

To review currently available literature regarding biology, risk factors, symptoms, pathogenesis, and therapeutics of uterine leiomyoma. Extensive literature review of 200 articles aiming towards uterine leiomyoma. Uterine leiomyomas are solid abdominal monoclonal tumours mostly develop in myometrium of uterus and adversely affect endometrium. Fibroids in uterus are major cause of morbidity in women. Uterine fibroids also show hereditary effects and reported in women of next generations. Submucosal and intramural fibroids distort uterine cavity, affect implantation and lead to infertility. Mechano-transduction from ECM components to intracellular components of myometrial cells stimulate cytoskeletal shape alterations and enhanced ECM stiffness provide basal node for tumour initiation. Oestrogen and progesterone further regulate development of uterine leiomyoma. Main aim of study is to distinguish uterine leiomyomas with higher efficacy to develop more effective medical treatment. Curcumin, EGCG and many more natural compounds may be considered as potential therapeutic agents and growth inhibitor for leiomyoma. Present review is focussed on biology. Risk factors, symptoms, pathogenesis and therapeutics of uterine leiomyoma. By regulating many cyclin dependent kinases (CDKs) and caspases, cell cycle checkpoints can be altered and fibroid growth be prevented. A comprehensive information has been obtained, although there are many lacunae and mechanism not so well understood. Yet present study may open new window for research for leiomyoma therapeutics.

Keywords: extracellular matrix, oestrogen, leiomyoma, natural products, progesterone, pathogenomics

1. Introduction

1.1 Search strategies

A comprehensive literature search was conducted spanning from the initial records up to May 15, 2023, by researchers. The search was executed across prominent databases including PubMed, Google Scholar, and Web of Science. The search strategy was structured into three distinct sections, incorporating Subject Headings terms along with relevant free-text terms related to Uterine leiomyoma, encompassing aspects of pathogenesis and therapeutics. Notably, no constraints were imposed on language, publication date, or any other limiting factors during the search process.

Uterine leiomyomas (known as uterine fibroids) are solid abdominal monoclonal tumours developing in myometrium of uterus and adversely affecting endometrium. Fibroids in uterus are major cause of morbidness in women. Leiomyomas are most common public health problem around world. Commonness of fibroid development in women is age-dependent and by an age of 50 years it has been detected in 80% of women. According to a WHO report, 6.6% of global women (nearly 235 million) population was affected of fibroids [1]. It is most commonly diagnosed in women with age of 30 and 40 years. 70–80% of women are affected by uterine fibroids during their lifetime by age of 50 [2]. 40-60% of all hysterectomies performed in Italy, 39% in United States, and 65% in India annually are indications of fibroids [3]. 30-50% women are symptomatic otherwise remaining detected incidentally by ultrasonography imaging [4]. Fibroid have shown 29% frequency of hospitalisation during 15–54 years of age [5].

In a general context, leiomyomas are comprised of a combination of smooth muscle cells, fibroblasts, and an interstitial matrix that includes constituents such as collagen, proteoglycan, and fibronectin. These elements form a complex structure characterised by the presence of interwoven bundles of lance-shaped or stellate myocytes. Notably, this arrangement exhibits minimal cellular pleomorphism or mitotic activity, as noted in Ref. [6]. The process of leiomyoma formation involves two main components: the alteration of normal smooth muscle cells into abnormal ones and their subsequent transformation into distinct tumour nodules [7]. Leiomyoma may be solitaire or multiple tumour nodules within same uterus surrounded by different quantity of interstitial fibrous connective mesodermal tissue. Leiomyomas development is directly influenced by increased exposure of steroid hormones. There is slow proliferation of fibroid myometrial cells with deposition of ECM (especially excessive collagen deposition) generally in steroid-hormone-dependent manner [8]. Size of fibroids can vary from large sized totally filling whole uterine cavity to small sized in millimetre, centimetres or microscopic [9].

Uterine fibroids are diagnosed by imaging ultrasonography, sonohysterography, X-ray examination, magnetic resonance imaging and by histological evaluation. Most common symptoms observed after uterine fibroids development are menorrhagia, pain in pelvic region, infertility, heavy bleeding during menstruation, anaemia, constipation, urine incontinence etc. [10]. Increased micturition, incontinence and obstruction of the ureter are symptoms associated with urinary tract. Blockage of the ureter, which can result in hydronephrosis, necessitates prompt treatment. Additionally, the presence of symptoms related to the gastrointestinal tract, such as constipation and tenesmus (characterised by the recurrent urge to defecate), can often be attributed to the development of fibroids [11].

Fibroids development in uterus results in distorted uterine cavity hence resulting in failure of implantation and pregnancy [12]. Pregnant women affected by fibroids experience a higher incidence of complications during pregnancy. These complications include preterm delivery (16.7% compared to 6.3%), premature rupture of membranes (14.3% compared to 2.1%), placental abruption (7.5% compared to 0.9%), foetal malformation (6.2% compared to 3.3%), postpartum haemorrhage (33% compared to 6%), and fatal malpresentation (19% compared to 4.4%), when compared to women who do not have fibroids [13]. Shoulder dystocia, postnatal bleeding, ectopic pregnancy, or miscarriage are other complaints associated with fibroid development during pregnancy. Fibroids represents 10% of infertility cases in women [14]. Symptoms severity and manifestation time directly depends on fibroids location in uterus. For example, when compared with subserosal fibroids, submucosal fibroids result in more irregular uterine bleeding and pregnancy problems [15].

Pre-menstruation, obesity, parity, fatty acids rich diet, smoking, caffeine and alcohol are some of risk factors for developing fibroid [5]. Fibroids can also develop to women having genomic syndromes like Alport syndrome, Cowden syndrome, reed syndrome etc. [16]. Uterine fibroids also show hereditary effects and most likely effects women of next generations.

Leiomyomas are of monoclonal origin i.e. originate from single myometrial cell. Two leiomyomas within a single uterus can vary in their molecular-genetical background. Identification of genetical mechanisms of leiomyoma concerning cellular differentiation of myocytes is still under research and not well known. But there are evidences of involvement of genes like oestrogen receptor (ER) gene, progesterone receptor (PR) gene, high mobility group (HMG) genes, fumarate hydratase (FH) gene, mediator sub-complex (MED) gene and collagen type-IV genes (COL4A and COL5A) which influences genomic instability [17]. Many genes in cell proliferation, differentiation and ECM production are dysregulated in uterine leiomyomas. These genes may be effectors or promoters of uterine leiomyomas growth. Regulation of gene expression is dependent on gonadal steroid hormones level variations during different phases of menstrual cycle. Fibroid develops between menarche and menopause [8]. Most fibroids shrink after menopause. Hysterectomy, myomectomy and uterine artery embolization are the commonest medical treatments used for curing fibroid development [18].

2. Risk factors

There are several exogenous and endogenous risk factors associated with uterine fibroids. These are age, race, early menarche, genetic factors, hormonal factors, stress, obesity and other factors such as diet rich in red meat, high blood pressure, hypertension, family history, caffeine intake etc.

2.1 Exogenous risk factors

2.1.1 Diet

Diet plays critical role in uterine fibroid development. Eating habits of different countries explain different frequencies of leiomyoma. Endogenous hormone metabolism gets modified due to variation in dietary components.

a. Dairy products: higher composition of fatty acids of animal origin increases risk of fibroid development rather than of dairy origin. Dairy product consumption decreases fibroid development risk in a dosage-dependent manner. A 33% decreased risk of fibroid development was observed in women with ≥4 intake of dairy product per day compared with those having no or less serving per day [19].

b. Red meat: red meats and beef consumption increase fibroids risk whereas fish consumption shows a decrease risk [20].

c. Fruits and vegetables: an inverse association is also observed in between uterine fibroids and high fruits and vegetable consumption especially tomatoes, apples, citrus fruits and cruciferous vegetable. These dietary components decrease risk of fibroid commonness by inhibiting rapid proliferation, programmed cell death and hormone dependency [21].

d. Vitamins: vitamin D supplemented diet also reduces fibroid development as vitamin D3 acts as an antitumor agent inhibiting cell proliferation [22]. Vitamin D3 also acts as an anti-estrogenic agent and reduces steroid hormone receptor expression making it a novel therapeutic option for uterine fibroid treatment [23]. An inverse relation has been observed in between Vitamin A derived from animal product and fibroid development [21]. Vitamin A gets transformed into more effective compounds like retinoic acid that shows inhibiting efficiency in leiomyoma expansion in vitro. No significant relationship has been observed in between Vitamin C and E dietary intake and fibroid risk [24].

2.1.2 Smoking

Smoking and uterine fibroid risk association are controversial [25]. Smoking reduces circulating oestrogen levels by inhibiting aromatase activity which is responsible for conversion of androgen to oestrogen, therefore decreasing oestrogen bioavailability [26]. In contrast, smoking also exerts oestrogen related effect on uterus promoting cell proliferation [27]. Therefore, effect of smoking on fibroid remains under conflict.

2.1.3 Alcohol

Alcohol increase fibroid development risk. BWHS examined risk association in regard to alcoholic beverage types [28]. An increased relationship of beer (having greater content of phytoestrogen) consumption has been found rather than in wine [25].

2.1.4 Caffeine

Huge coffee intake is a risk for younger women and not for women of all ages [20]. Caffeine intake stimulates early follicular phase oestradiol level [29] and also increases sex steroid production and phosphodiesterase inhibition [30]. Caffeine exerts negative effect only when consumed greater than 500 mg per day [31].

2.1.5 Endocrine disruptors

Endocrine Disruptor Chemicals (EDCs) present in pharmaceuticals, plasticizers especially DES (Diethylstilbestrol), dioxins, biphenyls, phthalates and organochlorines are sensitive to uterine fibroid development. High dioxin serum level shows a reduced fibroid risk [32]. DES increase tumorigenesis [33]. Mechanism of EDC exposer which increases tumorigenesis is quiet under research.

2.1.6 Exercise

Exercise induces a protective effect on fibroids. Women exercising regularly have lower risk of fibroids in comparison to those who do not do exercise [34]. Physical activity reduces sex steroid hormones circulation, insulin levels and availability of free circulating oestrogen by increasing SHBG levels. A reciprocal relationship between physical activities and fibroids presence has been observed [35]. This study also reveals a dose-dependent response i.e. women performing high level of physical exercise have less commonness level of fibroids then who performs fewer physical activities (≥7 h per week vs. <2 h per week). Benign uterine tumours develop 1.4 times more likely in non-athletic women than athletic women [25].

2.1.7 Stress

Stress plays important role in pathogenesis of uterine fibroids. Greater risk of fibroid development depends on larger count of vital life incidents and stress intensity [36]. The NHS II found a higher uterine leiomyoma prevalence in between women who are long-serving to ill-treat in their early-stages of life. The risk was lesser among women appearing in an emotionally supportive relationship in their teenage which recommend that the emotional and social support can diminish the influence of stress on risk [37].

2.2 Endogenous risk factors

2.2.1 Age

The primary and most significant risk factor for the development of uterine fibroids is age. The occurrence of leiomyomas has not been documented before adolescence, and their frequency diminishes notably after menopause [14]. With advancing age, the likelihood of developing fibroids significantly escalates, resulting in a substantial increase in both frequency and quantity of fibroids [38]. Moreover, the rate of hospitalisation due to uterine fibroids follows an age-related pattern. It reaches its highest point at 62.7 per 10,000 women within the age range of 45–49 years. Subsequently, this rate gradually declines to 31.8 per 10,000 women within the age range of 50–54 years [39].

2.2.2 Race

Lifetime risk for uterine fibroid (aggregated risk of fibroid development by 50 years of age) have been reported more in black women (78%) [14]. Black women develop fibroids 10 years before when compared to white women. The prevalence of uterine fibroids is noteworthy among different racial groups. Among African-American women, the occurrence of fibroids in the uterus reaches 60% by the age of 35, and this percentage rises to 80% by the age of 50. In contrast, white women have a lower incidence of fibroid development, with approximately 40% affected by age 35, which then increases to nearly 70% by age 50 [40]. Notably, uterine fibroids in black women are often characterised by being numerous and larger in size. Additionally, these fibroids tend to manifest more complex and severe symptoms in comparison to those experienced by white women [28].

2.2.3 Obesity

Obesity is considered as a risky factor for fibroids development in uterus. An increase in body mass index (BMI) is directly correlated with increased fibroid risk [34]. Risk increases 20% with every 10 kg increase of weight [41]. It may act through hormonal or through inflammatory mechanism. Obesity increases conversion rate of adrenal steroid hormones into oestrogen and reduces production of sex hormones binding globulin (SHBG) from hepatic cells, resultant being higher amount of free active oestrogen [34]. Fibroids presence in uterus was higher in case of visceral fat and peritoneal fat thickness. However, subcutaneous fat thickness does not show any significant association with fibroids presence [42].

2.2.4 Reproductive factors

a. Pregnancy and parity: pregnancy showed a protective effect on fibroid development. High parity (3 or more deliveries) decreases fibroid risk up to five times [43]. Growth of fibroid is affected by sharp elevation during very early pregnancy and decline postpartum period of oestrogen and progesterone. Fibroid that develops during first trimester of pregnancy get reduced in diameter by 0.5 cm. However high parity and less leiomyoma commonness are assumed over estimated as fibroid existence leads to infertility therefore reduces parity itself [31].

b. Early menarche: an inverse association was found in between early age menarche and fibroid risk [44]. Menarche at an early age i.e. before age of 10 years is associated with higher risk of developing fibroids. Early menarche is accompanied with increased oestradiol to post-pubertal levels which can probably lead to increase in fibroid growth [45]. This may describe that generally black patients have earlier menarche than in white patients which show that black patients have early onset of disease [46].

2.2.5 Family history

Uterine leiomyomas is a hereditary disease and tend to run in families. Family history of women with fibroids has been reported. Mutation in a single myometrial stem cell in uterus (existing from birth) is believed to be responsible for fibroid formation. Fibroid have monoclonal development i.e. arises from a single cell abnormality, but it is unknown what triggers the change from a normal to an aberrant myocyte [47, 48]. Numerous researches have shown that fibroid exhibit specified gene-directed chromosomal abnormalities [49]. Whatever causes the transition of a normal myocyte into an aberrant one, it is more frequent or more powerful in families where fibroids are more common, resulting in twice as many of these tumours as in families where fibroids are caused by somatic changes. Some fibroids may manifest as a result of inherited genes and so have a family frequency, whereas others may manifest as a result of acquired gene mutations [50].

2.2.6 Genetic factors

Fibroid growth and development is directly enhanced by genetic abnormalities. Whole genome sequencing and gene expression profiling of different uterine leiomyomas and neighbouring myometrium was performed [51]. MED12, HMGA2, FH and many other genomic abnormalities were observed which acts as genetic hits for uterine fibroid development. The accurate racial inconsistency in uterine leiomyoma commonness and increased familial aggregation of uterine fibroids specifies that molecular level factors are also basis of fibroid formation. Pathology data (especially in larger tumours) show non-random chromosomal abnormalities that are related to mutations in cell growth regulation. These chromosomal abnormalities are preceded due to clonal expansion of leiomyoma cells, indicating that chromosomal abnormalities also effects growth [52]. Familial aggregation of fibroids has been reported [53] and studies in mainly white women populations have reported cross-product ratios of 2.2–4 for female relative of women having leiomyoma to develop the condition [54].

3. Pathogenesis of uterine leiomyoma

The cellular origin of uterine fibroids remains a subject of ongoing debate and uncertainty within the scientific community. However, several studies provide support for the notion that each fibroid originates from the transformation of a single myometrial stem cell, driven by the influence of ovarian steroid hormones. These fibroids are considered monoclonal tumours, originating from a single cell with genetic alterations [55]. Human myometrial tissues comprise somatic cells exhibiting multipotent characteristics. Under the influence of ovarian hormones, these myometrial tissue cells engage in asymmetric division, leading to self-renewal and the generation of daughter cells responsible for tissue regeneration [56]. It's worth noting that fibroids in the human uterus possess fewer stem cells compared to normal myometrium. Interestingly, stem cells derived from fibroid tissue, as opposed to those from normal myometrium, are found to carry mutations in the MED12 gene (mediator complex subunit 12). This genetic alteration suggests a significant genetic event that transforms the myometrial stem cell, resulting in a coordinated interaction with neighbouring myometrial tissue and ultimately culminating in the formation of a fibroid tumour [57].

3.1 Mechano-transduction

Hormonal stimulation is an essential factor for tumour growth but non-hormonal factors such as hypoxia, repeated myometrial damage, repair and changes especially muscular contraction during pregnancy, childbirth and menstruation, chronic inflammation and extravasation of menstrual blood into myometrium may be responsible for fibroid initiation [58]. Chronic inflammation can also act as a major factor as it increases vascularization, vascular permeability and fibroblast proliferation [7]. Abnormal inflammatory response could be produced due to menstrual damage. Ischemic damage, resulting from reperfusion after ischemia in the myometrium, might be initiated by the contractions of the myometrium during menstrual bleeding. Cells within the myometrium that are affected by this damage could potentially transform into uterine fibroid progenitor cells. These cells may undergo apoptosis and be eliminated during the follicular phase, or if they manage to survive, they might develop mechanisms that shield them from oxidative stress and apoptosis, leading to their differentiation into uterine fibroid progenitor cells [59]. Frequent damage occurring within the myometrium and its adjacent extracellular matrix (ECM) components gives rise to a state of mechanical stress. The ECM plays a direct role in orchestrating irregularities in tumour composition, structural arrangement, fluid distribution, and firmness. Consequently, these aberrations escalate the mechanical stress encountered within the tissue. This escalated mechanical stress serves as a trigger for the transmission of mechanical signals (mechano-transduction) through collagen and other ECM constituents. These signals travel through transmembrane receptors, prompting modifications in cellular behaviour and the cytoskeletal framework. As a result, the heightened stiffness of the ECM further intensifies, setting the stage for the initiation of tumours by establishing a basal node in the process [60]. ECM components such as collagen, fibronectin and proteoglycans show abnormalities both qualitatively (altered and unordered composition) and quantitatively (two-fold excessive deposition) in uterine leiomyomas. These altered components act as a source for growth factors, cytokines, inflammatory and angiogenic mediators and proteases. Leiomyoma shows abnormal fibroblast structure and orientation. Focal adhesions get formed by clustering and activation of integrin receptors. This further leads to activation of FAK (focal adhesion kinases) which activate MAPK and PI3K pathways, altering cell cycle regulatory proteins and enhancing proliferation [61]. As compared to myometrium, type I and III collagen mRNA and type I and V collagen proteins are higher in fibroids. Both autocrine and paracrine processes regulate fibroid growth [7]. Uterine fibroids develop in between menarche and menopause. A lot of chances are present in between for any genetic hit to develop fibroid.

3.2 Initiation of tumour formation

Normal myometrial tissue containing pool of stem cells showing self-renewal ability and controls proliferation of normal myometrial myocytes under steroid hormone (oestrogen and progesterone) influence. Mature myocytes show much more oestrogen receptor α (ERα) and progesterone receptor (PR) expression then stem cells. So, sex hormones dependent cell proliferation is regulated by steroid hormone receptors present on these mature cells [62]. Self-renewal and proliferation of stem cells is induced by paracrine factors like WNT ligands, released from mature myocytes. Molecular strike like MED 12 mutation or chromosomal abnormality may changeover a myometrial stem cell into a fibroid stem cell [7]. Such fibroid cell with a genetic hit self-renews and divides in uncontrolled manner until differentiates into mature fibroid myocyte (**Figure 1**). Along with this, fibroid myocyte also gains other epigenetic and phenotypic anomalies. Steroid hormone receptors exhibit robust activity within mature fibroid myocytes, translating steroid hormone signals to stem cells through paracrine mechanisms. A solitary converted fibroid stem cell can initiate the development of a benign fibroid tumour characterised by well-defined boundaries, which progressively grows within the myometrial tissue. The creation of the extracellular matrix (ECM) also plays a role in facilitating the expansion of the tumour [63].

3.3 Growth of tumour

In vivo experiments reveal that human fibroid tumours growth require presence of multipotent somatic stem cells depending upon levels of oestrogen and progesterone. Fibroids stem cells as compared to myometrial cells express significantly small level of steroid hormones (oestrogen and progesterone) receptors. However, fibroid stem cells growth essentially requires myometrial cells along with excess levels of steroid receptors as well as their hormones i.e. oestrogen and progesterone. Oestrogen and progesterone action on leiomyoma stem cells is regulated by uterine

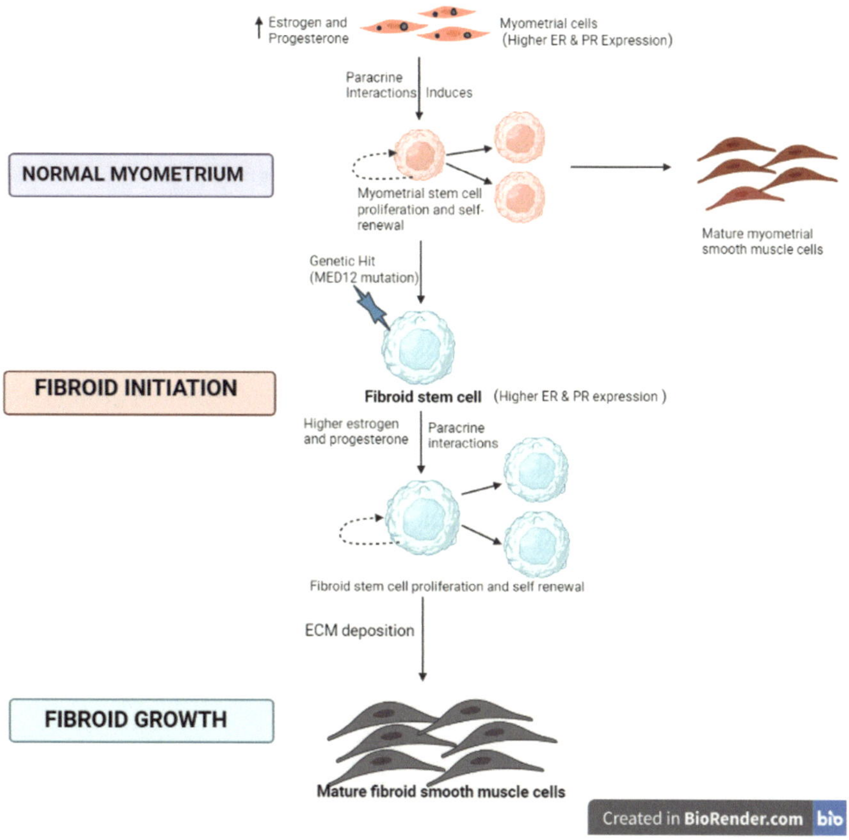

Figure 1.
Tumorigenesis of fibroids: normal myometrium contain stem cells for regeneration during menstruation, pregnancy etc. mature myometrium cells have higher levels of ER and PR expression than stem cells. After binding of oestrogen and progesterone to their respective receptors, they induce paracrine interactions to nearby stem cells and induces cell proliferation and self-renewal. Genetic alteration such as MED12 mutation transforms myometrial stem cell into fibroid stem cell. Many genetic and epigenetic changes stimulate their transformation. These fibroid cells self-renew and proliferate uncontrollably and at last differentiate into mature fibroid smooth muscle cell. ER and PR higher expression in mature fibroid-stem cells again paracrinely induces immature cells for division. ECM excessive deposition further contributes to tumour growth. In this way, single transformed fibroid stem cell forms fibroid tumour with well outlined boundaries. Courtesy by Bulun [63].

involuntary myometrial cells in paracrine fashion. This cell-to-cell vicinity interaction with neighbouring cells supports fibroid stem cells self-renewal [64]. Signalling by Wingless type protein (WNT)-β-catenin pathway effectively regulate somatic stem cell function in myometrium and uterine leiomyoma tissue. Almost similar levels of β-catenin were observed in myometrium and fibroid tissue [65]. But as effects of β-catenin are influenced at stem cells level, its level was not of much difference when compared to both myometrium and fibroid cells. Targeted depletion of β-catenin within the uterine myometrium leads to a reduction in uterine dimensions, accompanied by the replacement of uterine tissue with adipose cells. This process disrupts the usual course of myometrial differentiation or myocyte regeneration [56]. Conversely, an excessive presence of β-catenin in the uterine mesenchyme during the embryonic phase results in the emergence of tumours reminiscent of fibroids within the uterus [66]. WNT proteins get secreted and attach to cell-surface receptors of frizzled family, resulting in β-catenin decreased deterioration in cytosol by protein cascade activation. This leads to β-catenin amount variation reaching to nucleus. Due to this escaped degradation, cytoplasmic β-catenin enters nucleus and binds with chromatin and T-cell transcription factor (TCF) family proteins and regulates a number of gene expression and cellular functions like cell destiny, differentiation and tumorigenesis. Ovarian steroid hormone (oestrogen and progesterone) enhances WNT secretion from mature myocytes surrounding stem cells. WNT activates β-catenin-TCF pathway producing TGFβ in mature cells leading excessive ECM formation (**Figure 2**). MED12 mutation is linked to increased expression of TGFβ receptor activating its downstream signalling involving SMAD and MAPK mediating fibroid stem cell self-renewing and procreation [63]. Interfering with WNT binding or inhibiting β-catenin in leiomyoma stem-precursor cells has a notable effect in curtailing the expansion of tumours [67]. Activation of the WNT-β-catenin pathway spurs the expression of TGF-β3 (Transforming Growth Factor β3), which in turn triggers cell proliferation and the construction of extracellular matrix (ECM) components—particularly the ECM protein fibronectin—in human fibroid tissue, surpassing the levels observed in the myometrium [68]. This TGF-β3 derived from fibroid tissue curbs the expression of local anticoagulant factors within adjacent endomyocytes, consequently leading

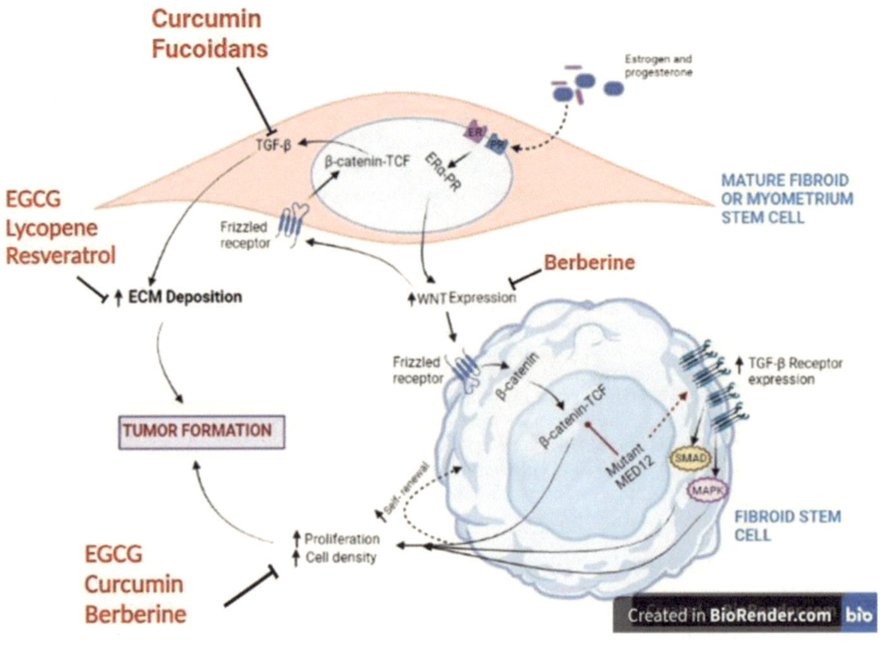

Figure 2.
Paracrine signalling among oestrogen and progesterone hormones, β-catenin-TGF-β pathways and MED12 in fibroid cells as well as potential role of natural products: oestrogen and progesterone binds to their respective receptors (higher expression) present on fibroid stem cells in paracrine way. This binding stimulates WNT secretion from mature myocytes. WNT further activates β-catenin-TCF pathway and stimulates TGF-β production in mature cells and resultantly excessive deposition. MED12 mutation in stem cells induces TGF-β increased expression and activates downstream signalling by activating SMAD and MAPK proteins enhancing self-renewal and procreation of cells. Natural compounds such as EGCG, lycopene, resveratrol (maintains ECM deposition and its protein formation in a regular manner), berberine, curcumin, fucoidans (suppress increased TGF-β and WNT expression in normal myometrium cells) inhibits myometrium stem cell conversion to fibroid stem cell and inhibits cell proliferation so regulating tumour growth (where TGF-β is transforming growth factor-β; MED12 is mediator subunit complex 12; WNT is wingless-related integration site protein, TCF is T-cell transcription factor, SMAD is mothers against decapentaplegic homologue protein and MAPK is mitogen-activated protein kinase). Courtesy by Bulun [63].

to prolonged menstrual bleeding—an indicator of its affiliation with fibroids. These findings underscore a significant interplay between the activation of the WNT-β-Catenin pathway, the TGF-β pathway, ovarian hormones, and stem cell renewal, culminating in the formation of uterine fibroid tumours [66].

4. Steroid hormones and receptors as main regulators of uterine leiomyoma development

A universal feature of uterine fibroids is its response towards oestrogen and progesterone. Oestrogen and progesterone and their receptors are key regulators of fibroid development.

4.1 Oestrogen and its receptor

Oestrogen simulates uterine fibroid growth through oestrogen receptors. Oestrogen receptors have two isoforms i.e. ERα and ERβ encoded by two different genes—ESR1 and ESR2 respectively, present on chromosome no. 6q25 and 14q23-24.1. ESR1 have eight exons spanning in more than 140 Kbps region. At boundary of intron 1 and exon 2 of ESR1, a well-known T/C SNP recognised by restriction enzyme Pvu II in uterine leiomyoma in South Indian population was revealed. This polymorphism also shows confirmed association in Asian Taiwanese, American and Hispanic population. It also shows association with other reproductive pathologies like ovulatory dysfunction, ovarian cysts, and breast cancer in women revealing its importance in affecting ER functionality [69]. ESR2 also have eight exons spanning in approximately 40 Kbps region. Two different promoters namely, 0 N and 0 K promoters initiate transcription of ESR2 gene. These transcription promoters (mainly 0 N) are involved in uterine leiomyoma pathogenesis as its variation alters ER-β protein levels. ESR2 gene polymorphisms reveal a significant association with uterine leiomyoma in South Indian population [8]. ER are of two types—nuclear and plasma membrane bound (mER and GPR30). 5–10% of total ERs are plasma membrane localised. ERα and ERβ, both isoforms are localised at plasma membrane [70]. By altering transcriptional activity and hastening signal transmission, oestrogen produces its effects. Oestrogen binds to nucleus ER and E_2-ER complex regulate transcriptional activities while mER are bounded with heat shock protein 90 (HSP90), also responsible for trafficking in nuclear materials. Binding of E_2 to mER results in HSP90 dissociation, dimerization of ER and other conformational changes, resulting in binding of ER to EREs of DNA at target genes promoters [71]. On other hand, E_2 binding on mER form homodimers which leads to activation of several kinases, like src which further activate PI3K and ERK pathways. GPR30 activation generates cAMP, Ca^{2+} release and activation of protein kinase and then transcriptional activation of some specific genes like c-fos, c-Jun etc. [72]. ERα and ERβ expression was noted in both myometrium and fibroid tissue [73]. Transcription is more dominantly activated by ERα and is stimulated by ERβ [74]. Fibroids shows enhanced oestrogen level than neighbouring myometrium and also enhanced aromatase and 17-β hydroxyl steroid dehydrogenase type1 levels [75]. Increased expression of aromatase also enhances fibroid tumorigenesis especially in black women. It has been observed that fibroid tissue from black women have high levels of aromatase than in white women resulting in increased levels of oestrogen in black women fibroid tissue [76]. Aromatase activity in fibroid cells locally increases oestrogen levels, along with it ovarian oestrogen level also get exposed to fibroid tissue [75]. Multiple promoters controlled by transcription factors in fibroid tissue stimulate single aromatase protein expression that transforms circulating steroid hormone precursors into oestrogen [77]. Fibroids are capable of producing sufficient oestrogen in a paracrine fashion to retain their auto-expansion. Gonadotrophin independent aromatase expression in fibroids is still unknown [78]. Aromatase inhibitors effectively shrink fibroid volume suggesting that aromatase inhibition is important regulatory mechanism in fibroid shrinkage [79]. Aromatase RNA expression was not observed in myometrium without fibroids [75]. ERα and ERβ expression in uterine leiomyoma leads to differentiation of fibroid precursor cells [73]. Oestrogen binding to ERα functions in a permissive way enabling tissue to react towards progesterone by enhancing PR expression. Oestrogen increases multiple growth factor, collagen (ESM component), oestrogen receptor and progesterone receptor expression in fibroid pathogenesis [80]. Oestrogen rapidly activates different kind of kinases [81]. Oestrogen stimulates fibroid cells proliferation by ATP-sensitive potassium channels opening. Oestrogen stimulates fibroid expansion by suppressing normal p53 functions [62]. Leiomyoma proliferation requires oestrogen, however it is not adequate on its own [78]. Oestrogen and its receptor, ERα, play a pivotal role in controlling the expression of PR. Notably, oestrogen alone does not function as a mitogen in vivo [62]. Leiomyoma proliferative activity increases with combined oestrogen and progesterone level in postmenopausal women but does not show enhancement alone with oestrogen replacement [82]. Disruption of oestrogen signalling pathway with ERα mutant decreases wild type ERα and PR gene expression [83].

4.2 Progesterone and its receptor

Progesterone is primary maintainer of fibroid extension and volume maintenance while oestrogen mainly induces PR expression [62]. Progesterone shows its effects through progesterone receptors. Progesterone gene receptor (PGR) gene has two isoforms i.e. PR-A and PR-B located on chromosome 11q22-23. Two different promoters transcribe these two isoforms but have same translational site except that PR-B have an additional 165 amino acids [84]. Progesterone acts through PR-A and PR-B showing enhanced level in fibroids in comparison to myometrium [85]. Leiomyoma surfaces exhibit heightened expression of PR-B mRNA. It's important to note that PR-A is primarily involved in ovulation and governs the anti-proliferative impacts of progesterone within the uterus. On the other hand, PR-B plays a crucial role in the typical development and operation of mammary glands [86] Progesterone and PR were necessary and sufficient for fibroid expansion, as they stimulate cell proliferation, interstitial matrix deposition and cellular hypertrophy [87]. Progesterone receptors are also of two types—nuclear and membrane bound. mPR have three isoforms—mPRα, mPRβ and mPRγ [88]. Pg bounded PR binds at progesterone response elements on DNA and regulates transcription of several genes. PR have proline-rich motif that directly activate ERK-MAPK signalling pathway [89]. It also activates AKT and glycogen synthase kinase-3B (GSK3B). This shows that progesterone stimulates leiomyoma cells proliferation by activating AKT signalling pathway. Secretory phase of menstrual cycle (which is progesterone dominant) shows higher mitotic activity than proliferative phase (which is oestrogen dominant) [70]. ER are activated by PR-B type while suppressed by PR-A type [84]. The progesterone receptor, a transcription factor activated by its ligand (progesterone or anti-progestins), serves as a master regulator of gene expression, overseeing the effects of progesterone and anti-progestins on a multitude of genes [90]. Anti-progestins like RU486

(Mifepristone) bound with PR co-relates with more than 7000 DNA sites and genes encoding in these regions controls cell growths, focal adhesion and ECM functioning [91]. Anti-progestin bounded PR in fibroid cells assembles a transcriptional complex forming bridge between DNA sequence and transcription starts sites of KLF11 (Kruppel-like transcription factor 11) resulting in KLF11 gene and protein expression. In response, KLF11 inhibits fibroid cell proliferation. KLF11 (tumour suppressor gene) is a transcription factor interacts with PR signalling and thus with fibroid cell proliferation [92]. In contrast, progesterone bound PR maintains KLF11 transcriptional repression by same DNA sequence regulation resulting in increased cell proliferation of fibroid. On other hand, progesterone binding to PR increases apoptotic inhibitory BCL2 (B-cell lymphoma 2) protein level by binding with a DNA sequence proximate upstream of BCL2 transcription start site and therefore decreasing apoptosis in fibroid tissue [63].

Both progesterone and oestrogen exert control over growth factors and their corresponding signalling pathways [93]. The activation of steroid hormone receptors leads to the upregulation of growth factors and receptor tyrosine kinases (RTKs), which subsequently operate through the mitogen-activated protein kinase (MAPK) cascade. This intricate process mediates various cellular functions, including transcription, translation, and cell proliferation [94]. Also, progesterone binding to cytoplasmic PR speedily activate extra-nuclear phosphatidylinositol-3-kinase-AKT signalling pathway which increases fibroid cell proliferation and inhibits apoptosis [89]. These two sex hormones interactions with other transcription factors were intricate. Progesterone also shows non-genomic actions such as AKT pathway activation promoting tumour expansion by cell survival stimulation and programmed cell death inhibition [89]. Progesterone upregulate EGF and TGFβ3 expression [68] and LAT-2 level i.e. L-type amino acid transporter-2 and downregulates TNFα expression and IGF1 expression through PR-B while PR-A upregulate it [95]. Progesterone is a more significant regulator of fibroid expansion than oestrogen, according to progesterone receptor modulators (PRMs), which are therapeutically utilised to treat leiomyoma [96].

5. Natural products as therapeutic agents for uterine leiomyoma

Now-a-days studies are focused from steroid hormones affect to fibroid stem cells and genetic abnormalities finding which will result in discoveries of new therapeutic agents like curcumin, green tea, resveratrol, lycopene and fucoidans (**Table 1**).

5.1 Epigallocatechin gallate (EGCG)

Catechins make up 30–42% of the dry weight of the solids in green tea [111]. Epigallocatechin-3-gallate (EGCG), epigallocatechin (EGC), epicatechin-3-gallate (ECG), and epicatechin are the four main catechins found in green tea. Catechins are a class of bioflavonoids with anti-inflammatory and antioxidant properties [97]. By altering signalling pathways related to cell proliferation, transformation, infection sensitivity, and oxidative stress, EGCG prevents the growth of uterine fibroids tumours at every stage [88]. EGCG suppress proliferation of Human fibroid cell and enhance programmed cell death. EGCG effectively prevents UF cell proliferation by down-regulating cyclin dependent kinases (CDKs), including CDK2 and CDK4, initiating apoptosis and prevent angiogenesis [98]. Therefore, EGCG may be used as potential future therapeutic agent for fibroid treatment.

Natural products	Function	References
EGCG	Antioxidant; apoptosis initiation; angiogenesis prevention; CDKs[a] downregulation	Chung et al. [97]; Ahmed et al. [98]
Curcumin	Strong antioxidant; strong anti-inflammatory agent; stimulates apoptosis; inhibits excessive ECM deposition; decreases TGF[b]-β related signalling	Chung et al. [97]; Khan et al. [88]; Tsuiji et al. [99]
Vitamin D	Anti-fibrotic agent; decreases PCNA,[c] CDKs, BCL-2[d] expression	Halder et al. [100]
Berberine	Decreases HCG effect on leiomyoma cells; increases COX2[e] and PTTG1[f] expression	Lee et al. [101]; Wu et al. [102]
Resveratrol	Anti-oxidant; anti-tumour agent; decreases MMP-2[g], BCL-2, Caspase-3 & 9 expression and Akt[h] phosphorylation; increases expression of p21 and Bax	Salehi et al. [103]; Wu et al. [88]; Ho et al. [104]; Li et al. [105]
Fucoidans	Decreases fibronectin, collagen, vimentin, connective tissue growth factor; inhibits TGF-1 related signalling	Collins et al. [106]; Charboneau et al. [107]; Li et al. [108]
Lycopene	Shields cell from DNA damage; inhibits cell proliferation and differentiation; alter cell-cycle regulatory protein phosphorylation	Gajowik et al. [109]; Rao et al. [110]

[a]*CDKs—cyclin dependent kinases.*
[b]*TGF—transforming growth factor.*
[c]*PCNA—proliferating cell nuclear antigen.*
[d]*BCL2—B-cell lymphoma-2.*
[e]*COX2—cyclooxygenase-2.*
[f]*PTTG1—pituitary tumour transforming gene 1 protein.*
[g]*MMP-2—matrix metallopeptidase-9.*
[h]*Akt—protein kinase B.*

Table 1.
Natural products as potential therapeutic agent in uterine leiomyoma prevention.

5.2 Curcumin

The primary naturally occurring polyphenol in rhizome of curcuma longa is yellow-coloured curcumin. Curcumin has a number of beneficial qualities, including antimicrobial, anti-inflammatory, anti-tumorigenic, and anti-mutagenic. Curcumin reduces endothelial cell fibrosis and inhibits TGF-related endothelial-to-mesenchymal transition. Curcumin has a suppressive outcome on leiomyoma cell procreation and ECM buildup [97]. Curcumin induces apoptosis by regulating key factors such as extracellular signal-regulated kinases (ERKs), caspase-3, caspase-9, and nuclear factor kappa-light-chain-enhancer of activated B cells (NF-κB). Additionally, curcumin exerts inhibitory effects on processes within the extracellular matrix (ECM), dampening the proliferation of leiomyoma cells. This action is facilitated through the activation of peroxisome proliferator-activated receptor-γ (PPAR-γ) [99]. Notably, curcumin possesses robust antioxidant and anti-inflammatory properties, contributing to the maintenance of stable levels of fibronectin, collagen, tumour necrosis factor-α (TNF-α), interleukin-6 (IL-6), and vascular endothelial growth factor [88].

5.3 Vitamin D

Vitamin D acts as an anti-fibrotic agent, effectively diminishing the expression of key factors like proliferating cell nuclear antigen (PCNA), cyclin-dependent kinase 1 (CDK1), B-cell lymphoma 2 (BCL-2), and catechol-O-methyl transferase (COMT). This orchestrated suppression hinders cell proliferation and encourages programmed cell death within cultured human fibroid cells [100]. Total serum level of 1, 25-dihydroxyvitamin D3 and 25-hydroxyvitamin D3 was less in fibroids compared to myometrium of uterus in healthy women [112]. There is a dose-dependent response and an inverse correlation between the severity of uterine fibroids and serum vitamin D levels. So, vitamin D and their analogues can be used as a novel option for uterine fibroids treatment [113].

5.4 Berberine

A perennial herb *Scutellaria barbata* contains a plant-based alkaloid Berberine. Plants high in berberine lessen the effect of human chorionic gonadotrophin (HCG) on the proliferation of UF and myometrial cells [101]. Berberine blocks proliferation of uterine leiomyoma cells induced by oestrogen and progesterone as well as cell apoptosis, by keeping human normal uterine myometrium unaffected [114]. Uterine leiomyoma cells have cyclooxygenase-2 (COX2) and pituitary tumour transforming gene 1 protein (PTTG1) higher expression as compared to myometrium. It has been observed that berberine diminishes expression of both COX2 and PTTG1 [102]. There by indicates berberine as an antifibroid alkaloid.

5.5 Resveratrol

Red wines and several plant species contain resveratrol, a stilbenoid polyphenol. Resveratrol has strong anti-tumour and antioxidant properties [103]. Resveratrol inhibits ECM-related proteins like fibronectin, collagen types 1 and 3, fibromodulin, and biglycan expression. Additionally, resveratrol decreases expression of MMP-9 while increasing expression of tissue inhibitor of metalloproteinase 2 (TIMP2) protein in leiomyoma cells [115]. Resveratrol blocks the procreation of UF cells via the integrin v3 pathway. Pro-apoptotic gene p21 expression is increased by resveratrol, while anti-apoptotic gene expression is decreased. Resveratrol prevents Akt phosphorylation in uterine leiomyoma cells [104]. Resveratrol has an anti-proliferative and apoptotic effect on human cervical cancer cells by upregulating Bax expression, downregulating Bcl-2 proteins, and activating caspase-3 and -9 [105]. Resveratrol can be considered as therapeutic agent for leiomyoma.

5.6 Fucoidans

Highly sulphated polysaccharides known as fucoidans are present in a number of types of brown seaweed and brown algae. The type of carbohydrates, the amount of sulphates, and the molecular weight, all affect activity of fucoidans [106]. Although gamma-irradiated fucoidans exhibited stronger cell transformation inhibition, low molecular weight fucoidans possess to have greater cytotoxicity in cancer cell lines than natural fucoidan [107]. Fucoidans reduce the expression of fibronectin and connective tissue growth factor in fibrotic cells and also blocks TGF-1-induced epithelial-mesenchymal transition (EMT) [108]. In lungs, fucoidans blocks the ERK pathway to prevent the TGF-β1-related epithelial-mesenchymal transition [116]. According to a study, fucoidan induces cell growth reduction and lower the levels of the protein fibronectin, vimentin, α-SMA, and collagen. This organic compound reduced the translocation of β-catenin as well as the Smad2 and ERK1/2 pathways in this model [117] and has the potential of prevention of uterine leiomyoma.

5.7 Lycopene

Lycopene is a phytonutrient found in eatables including oranges, tomatoes, carrots, papaya, and watermelon that belong to the carotenoid family. The well-known antioxidant property of carotenoids shields cells from DNA damage, abnormal cell proliferation, and abnormal cell differentiation [109]. Incorporating lycopene into one's diet has been associated with a reduced risk of gastrointestinal, prostate, breast, and lung cancer development [118]. Consuming β-carotene raises the risk of uterine fibroid, but only in women who smoke. Lycopene modulates anti-tumour immunity and has an anti-proliferative effect in part by altering the synthesis of cell cycle-regulating proteins [110]. Lycopene can be well tested as therapeutic compound for treatment of leiomyoma.

These natural therapeutic compounds have potential to suppress pathogenesis and growth of fibroid tumour by regulating cell signalling pathways, regulating cell proliferation and apoptosis such as TGF-β-WNT-catenin pathway, PI3K-Akt pathway and MAPK-ERK pathway. Curcumin and fucoidans specifically suppress TGF-β expression and berberine regulate WNT expression. These three suppress dysregulated TGF-β-WNT-catenin signalling pathway. Apart from these, EGCG, lycopene and resveratrol regulate ECM proteins formation such as fibronectin, collagen, globulin etc. and ECM excessive deposition. They also reduce irregular ECM intercellular skeletal changes, suppress initiation of basal node and resultantly stop tumour initiation. EGCG, curcumin and berberine also check excessive cellular proliferation and increased cell density, thereby reduce excessive fibroid growth. These natural compounds alter signalling pathways related to cell proliferation, transformation, as well as oxidative stress. Further by regulating many cyclin dependent kinases (CDKs), caspases these natural compounds alter cell cycle checkpoints and ceases more cell proliferation (**Figure 2**). Natural therapeutic compounds with anti-tumour properties are potential agents for uterine fibroid prevention and management. Understanding the role of natural products in pathogenesis of fibroid development will open a new window for clinician to treat uterine fibroid. It is quiet important to distinguish uterine leiomyomas with higher efficacy and developing more effective medical treatment to prevent necessity of hysterectomy, myomectomy, or UAE surgeries.

6. Conclusion

Uterine leiomyomas are benign monoclonal tumours that originate in the myometrium and can impact the endometrium negatively. They very rarely undergo malignant transformation. The formation of a leiomyoma entails the transition of normal smooth muscle cells into abnormal ones, followed by the growth and proliferation of these transformed myocytes, culminating in the development of a tumour.

These leiomyomas are prevalent in approximately 80% of women of reproductive age. Common symptoms and indications of leiomyomas encompass irregular menstrual bleeding, pelvic pain, pelvic pressure, anaemia, infertility, and a tendency towards early pregnancy loss. Age, African-American race, obesity, less physical activity, malnutrition diet, alcohol and caffeine increase risk of fibroid development. Submucosal and intramural fibroids distort uterine cavity, affect implantation and leads to infertility. Alterations in genes such as MED12, HMGA2 and signalling pathways such as WNT-β-catenin stimulates uterine fibroid development. Oestrogen and progesterone along with their receptors are major mediators of fibroid growth. Due to their monoclonal origin, heterogeneity was observed in leiomyoma. Tumour within same uterus can be controlled by different genetic mechanism while two non-related patients can have same genetic defects.

Until today, major studies on fibroids concentrate on the involvement of steroid hormones in the formation of fibroid tumours. This results in development of medical treatment options like GnRH agonist, aromatase inhibitor and anti-progestins targeting theses steroid hormones. But no medical treatment was found that permanently shrink tumour or prevents its formation. Natural compounds such as EGCG, curcumin, vitamin D, lycopene, resveratrol have potential to alter signalling pathways related to cell proliferation, transformation, infection sensitivity, and oxidative stress. Regulation of cyclin dependent kinases (CDKs) and caspases alter cell cycle checkpoints and cease more cell proliferation (**Figure 2**). Efficacy and potential of natural compound as therapeutic agent is evident and a open window for future research in prevention and management of uterine leiomyoma.

Acknowledgements

CSIR is acknowledged for financial assistance to research scholar Sonia Narwal (CSIR-SRF).

Conflict of interest

The authors declare that they have no conflict of interest.

Notes

Sonia Narwal has nothing to disclose. Minakshi Vashist has nothing to disclose. Rohit Kaushik has nothing to disclose. Vandana Kalra has nothing to disclose. Reetu Hooda has nothing to disclose. Sunita Singh has nothing to disclose.

Author details

Sonia Narwal[1], Minakshi Vashist[1*], Rohit Kaushik[1], Vandana Kalra[2], Reetu Hooda[3] and Sunita Singh[4]

1 Department of Genetics, M. D. University, Rohtak, Haryana, India

2 Goswami Ganesh Dutta Sanatan Dharma College, Palwal, Haryana, India

3 Department of Gynaecology and Obstetrics, P.G.I.M.S., Rohtak, Haryana, India

4 Department of Pathology, P.G.I.M.S., Rohtak, Haryana, India

*Address all correspondence to: mvashist14@mdurohtak.ac.in

References

[1] Aninye IO, Laitner MH, Society for Women's Health Research Uterine Fibroids Working Group. Uterine fibroids: Assessing unmet needs from bench to bedside. Journal of Women's Health. 2021;**30**(8):1060-1067

[2] Ciebiera M, Włodarczyk M, Zgliczyński S, Łoziński T, Walczak K, Czekierdowski A. The role of miRNA and related pathways in pathophysiology of uterine fibroids—From bench to bedside. International Journal of Molecular Sciences. 2020;**21**(8):3016

[3] Shekhar C, Paswan B, Singh A. Prevalence, sociodemographic determinants and self-reported reasons for hysterectomy in India. Reproductive Health. 2019;**16**(1):1-6

[4] Giuliani E, As-Sanie S, Marsh EE. Epidemiology and management of uterine fibroids. International Journal of Gynecology & Obstetrics. 2020;**149**(1):3-9

[5] Pavone D, Clemenza S, Sorbi F, Fambrini M, Petraglia F. Epidemiology and risk factors of uterine fibroids. Best Practice & Research Clinical Obstetrics & Gynaecology. 2018;**46**:3-11

[6] Laganà AS, Vergara D, Favilli A, La Rosa VL, Tinelli A, Gerli S, et al. Epigenetic and genetic landscape of uterine leiomyomas: A current view over a common gynecological disease. Archives of Gynecology and Obstetrics. 2017;**296**(5):855-867

[7] Botía CP, Camarasa SC, Baixauli FR, Sanchez AC. Uterine fibroids: Understanding their origins to better understand their future treatments. Journal of Tumor Research. 2017;**3**(130):2

[8] Bharathi C, Anupama D, Pratibha N, Venkateshwari A. Impact of genetic variants in estrogen receptor-β gene in the etiology of uterine leiomyomas. Journal of Reproduction & Infertility. 2019;**20**(3):151

[9] Dvorská D, Braný D, Danková Z, Halašová E, Višňovský J. Molecular and clinical attributes of uterine leiomyomas. Tumor Biology. 2017;**39**(6):1010428317710226

[10] Stewart EA, Cookson CL, Gandolfo RA, Schulze-Rath R. Epidemiology of uterine fibroids: A systematic review. BJOG: An International Journal of Obstetrics & Gynaecology. 2017;**124**(10):1501-1512

[11] Lim WH, Cohen SC, Lamaro VP. Intra-abdominal haemorrhage from uterine fibroids: A systematic review of the literature. BMC Surgery. 2020;**20**(1):1-7

[12] Makker A, Goel MM, Nigam D, Mahdi AA, Das V, Agarwal A, et al. Aberrant Akt activation during implantation window in infertile women with intramural uterine fibroids. Reproductive Sciences. 2018;**25**(8):1243-1253

[13] Gupta SK. To determine the association between uterine leiomyomas and various maternal and fetal complications occurring during pregnancy, delivery and puerperium. International Journal of Life Sciences, Biotechnology and Pharma Research. 2023;**12**(2):833-839

[14] Murji A, Bedaiwy M, Singh SS, Bougie O. CAPTURE Registry Steering Committee. Influence of ethnicity on clinical presentation and quality of life

in women with uterine fibroids: Results from a prospective observational registry. Journal of Obstetrics and Gynaecology Canada. 2020;**42**(6):726-733

[15] Ricci G, Scrimin F, Sartore A, Borelli M, Zito G, Romano F, et al. Characteristics of submucous myomas and the risk of anemia. Medicina. 2022;**58**(11):1652

[16] Gundlapally J. Genetics behind uterine fibroids. Helix-The Scientific Explorer, Peer Reviewed Bimonthly International Journal. 2022;**12**(2):8-12

[17] Moyo MB, Parker JB, Chakravarti D. Altered chromatin landscape and enhancer engagement underlie transcriptional dysregulation in MED12 mutant uterine leiomyomas. Nature Communications. 2020;**11**(1): 1-6

[18] De La Cruz MS, Buchanan EM. Uterine fibroids: Diagnosis and treatment. American Family Physician. 2017;**95**(2):100-107

[19] Orta OR, Terry KL, Missmer SA, Harris HR. Dairy and related nutrient intake and risk of uterine leiomyoma: A prospective cohort study. Human Reproduction. 2020;**35**(2):453-463

[20] Tinelli A, Vinciguerra M, Malvasi A, Andjić M, Babović I, Sparić R. Uterine fibroids and diet. International Journal of Environmental Research and Public Health. 2021;**18**(3):1066

[21] Wise LA, Wesselink AK, Bethea TN, Brasky TM, Wegienka G, Harmon Q, et al. Intake of lycopene and other carotenoids and incidence of uterine leiomyomata: A prospective ultrasound study. Journal of the Academy of Nutrition and Dietetics. 2021;**121**(1):92-104

[22] Kumari R, Nath B, Gaikwad HS, Sharma M. Association between serum vitamin D level and uterine fibroid in premenopausal women in Indian population. Drug Discoveries & Therapeutics. 2022;**16**(1):8-13

[23] Vergara D, Catherino WH, Trojano G, Tinelli A. Vitamin D: Mechanism of action and biological effects in uterine fibroids. Nutrients. 2021;**13**(2):597

[24] Szydłowska I, Nawrocka-Rutkowska J, Brodowska A, Marciniak A, Starczewski A, Szczuko M. Dietary natural compounds and vitamins as potential cofactors in uterine fibroids growth and development. Nutrients. 2022;**14**(4):734

[25] Wesselink AK, Wegienka G, Coleman CM, Geller RJ, Harmon QE, Upson K, et al. A prospective ultrasound study of cigarette smoking and uterine leiomyomata incidence and growth. American Journal of Obstetrics and Gynecology. 2023;**229**(2):151.e1-151.e8

[26] Noble LS, Ramirez D. Role of aromatase inhibitors (AIs) and selective estrogen receptor modulators (SERMs) in the treatment of uterine leiomyoma. In: Uterine Fibroids. Obstetrics, Gynecology and women's Health. Oxfordshire, UK: Taylor & Francis Group - CRC Press; 2020. pp. 71-74

[27] Helle J, Keiler AM, Zierau O, Dörfelt P, Vollmer G, Lehmann L, et al. Effects of the aryl hydrocarbon receptor agonist 3-methylcholanthrene on the 17β-estradiol regulated mRNA transcriptome of the rat uterus. The Journal of Steroid Biochemistry and Molecular Biology. 2017;**171**:133-143

[28] Song S, Park S, Song BM, Lee JE, Cha C, Park HY. Risk of uterine

leiomyomata with menstrual and reproductive factors in premenopausal women. BMC Women's Health. 2023;**23**(1):1-10

[29] Ihenacho U, Sriprasert I, Mack WJ, Hamilton AS, Unger JB, Press MF, et al. A systematic review and meta-analysis of smoking and circulating sex hormone levels among premenopausal women. Nicotine and Tobacco Research. 2022;**24**(11):1705-1713

[30] Barcelos RP, Lima FD, Carvalho NR, Bresciani G, Royes LF. Caffeine effects on systemic metabolism, oxidative-inflammatory pathways, and exercise performance. Nutrition Research. 2020;**80**:1-7

[31] Coutinho LM, Assis WA, Spagnuolo-Souza A, Reis FM. Uterine fibroids and pregnancy: How do they affect each other? Reproductive Sciences. 2022;**29**(8):2145-2151

[32] Wise LA. Environmental chemicals and risk of uterine leiomyomata. In: Uterine Fibroids. 6000 Broken Sound Parkway NW, Suite 300, Boca Raton, FL 33487-2742: CRC Press; 2020. pp. 4-14

[33] Katz TA, Yang Q, Treviño LS, Walker CL, Al-Hendy A. Endocrine-disrupting chemicals and uterine fibroids. Fertility and sterility. 2016;**106**(4):967-977

[34] Wise LA, Laughlin-Tommaso SK. Epidemiology of uterine fibroids–From menarche to menopause. Clinical Obstetrics and Gynecology. 2016;**59**(1):2

[35] Karamihamidabad Z, Azima S, Najib F, Akbarzadeh M. Association of body mass index & android obesity with uterine leiomyoma among premenopausal women: A case–control study. Journal of Experimental and Clinical Medicine. 2022;**39**(4):1235-1240

[36] Kumari P, Kundu J. Prevalence, socio-demographic determinants, and self-reported reasons for hysterectomy and choice of hospitalization in India. BMC Women's Health. 2022;**22**(1):514

[37] Chiuve SE, Huisingh C, Petruski- Ivleva N, Owens C, Kuohung W, Wise LA. Uterine fibroids and incidence of depression, anxiety and self-directed violence: A cohort study. Journal of Epidemiology and Community Health. 2022;**76**(1):92-99

[38] Stewart EA, Laughlin-Tommaso SK, Levine D. Uterine fibroids (leiomyomas): Epidemiology, clinical features, diagnosis, and natural history. UpToDate. 2019;**3**:22

[39] Wright JD, Huang Y, Li AH, Melamed A, Hershman DL. Nationwide estimates of annual inpatient and outpatient hysterectomies performed in the United States. Obstetrics & Gynecology. 2022;**139**(3):446-448

[40] Harmon QE. The burden of uterine fibroids: A search for primary and secondary prevention. Fertility and Sterility. 2019;**111**(1):50-51

[41] Kwas K, Nowakowska A, Fornalczyk A, Krzycka M, Nowak A, Wilczyński J, et al. Impact of contraception on uterine fibroids. Medicina. 2021;**57**(7):717

[42] Ciavattini A, Delli Carpini G, Moriconi L, Clemente N, Orici F, Boschi AC, et al. The association between ultrasound-estimated visceral fat deposition and uterine fibroids: An observational study. Gynecological Endocrinology. 2017;**33**(8):634-637

[43] Sato F, Mori M, Nishi M, Kudo R, Miyake H. Familial aggregation of uterine myomas in Japanese women. Journal of Epidemiology. 2002;**12**(3):249-253

[44] Freytag D, Günther V, Maass N, Alkatout I. Uterine fibroids and infertility. Diagnostics. 2021;**11**(8):1455

[45] Adawe M, Sezalio M, Kanyesigye H, Kajabwangu R, Okello S, Bajunirwe F, et al. Prevalence, clinical presentation and factors associated with uterine fibroids among women attending the Gynecology Outpatient Department at a large referral Hospital in Southwestern Uganda. East Africa Science. 2022;**4**(1):48-53

[46] Yang Q, Ciebiera M, Bariani MV, Ali M, Elkafas H, Boyer TG, et al. Comprehensive review of uterine fibroids: Developmental origin, pathogenesis, and treatment. Endocrine Reviews. 2022;**43**(4):678-719

[47] Townsend DE, Sparkes R, Baluda MC, McClelland G. Unicellular histogenesis of uterine leiomyomas as determined by electrophoresis of glucose-6-phosphate dehydrogenase. American Journal of Obstetrics and Gynecology. 1970;**107**(8):1168-1173

[48] Hashimoto K, Azuma C, Kamiura S, Kimura T, Nobunaga T, Kanai T, et al. Clonal determination of uterine leiomyomas by analyzing differential inactivation of the X-chromosome-linked phosphoglycerokinase gene. Gynecologic and Obstetric Investigation. 1995;**40**(3):204-208

[49] Styer AK, Rueda BR. The epidemiology and genetics of uterine leiomyoma. Best Practice & Research Clinical Obstetrics & Gynaecology. 2016;**34**:3-12

[50] Machado-Lopez A, Simón C, Mas A. Molecular and cellular insights into the development of uterine fibroids. International Journal of Molecular Sciences. 2021;**22**(16):8483

[51] Mehine M, Mäkinen N, Heinonen HR, Aaltonen LA, Vahteristo P. Genomics of uterine leiomyomas: Insights from high-throughput sequencing. Fertility and Sterility. 2014;**102**(3):621-629

[52] Goad J, Rudolph J, Zandigohar M, Tae M, Dai Y, Wei JJ, et al. Single-cell sequencing reveals novel cellular heterogeneity in uterine leiomyomas. Human Reproduction. 2022;**37**(10):2334-2349

[53] Gross KL, Morton CC. Genetics and the development of fibroids. Clinical Obstetrics and Gynecology. 2001;**44**(2):335-349

[54] Vikhlyaeva EM, Khodzhaeva ZS, Fantschenko ND. Familial predisposition to uterine leiomyomas. International Journal of Gynecology & Obstetrics. 1995;**51**(2):127-131

[55] Linder D, Gartler SM. Glucose-6-phosphate dehydrogenase mosaicism: Utilization as a cell marker in the study of leiomyomas. Science. 1965;**150**(3692):67-69

[56] Arango NA, Szotek PP, Manganaro TF, Oliva E, Donahoe PK, Teixeira J. Conditional deletion of β-catenin in the mesenchyme of the developing mouse uterus results in a switch to adipogenesis in the myometrium. Developmental Biology. 2005;**288**(1):276-283

[57] Ono M, Qiang W, Serna VA, Yin P, Coon JS, Navarro A, et al. Role of stem cells in human uterine leiomyoma growth. PLoS One. 2012;**7**(5):e36935

[58] Baranov VS, Osinovskaya NS, Yarmolinskaya MI. Pathogenomics of uterine fibroids development. International Journal of Molecular Sciences. 2019;**20**(24):6151

[59] Islam MS, Protic O, Stortoni P, Grechi G, Lamanna P, Petraglia F, et al. Complex networks of multiple factors in the pathogenesis of uterine leiomyoma. Fertility and Sterility. 2013;**100**(1):178-193

[60] Leppert PC, Catherino WH, Segars JH. A new hypothesis about the origin of uterine fibroids based on gene expression profiling with microarrays. American Journal of Obstetrics and Gynecology. 2006;**195**(2):415-420

[61] Koohestani F, Braundmeier AG, Mahdian A, Seo J, Bi J, Nowak RA. Extracellular matrix collagen alters cell proliferation and cell cycle progression of human uterine leiomyoma smooth muscle cells. PLoS One. 2013;**8**(9):e75844

[62] Ali M, Ciebiera M, Vafaei S, Alkhrait S, Chen HY, Chiang YF, et al. Progesterone signaling and uterine fibroid pathogenesis; molecular mechanisms and potential therapeutics. Cell. 2023;**12**(8):1117

[63] Bulun SE. Uterine fibroids. New England Journal of Medicine. 2013;**369**(14):1344-1355

[64] Mas A, Cervelló I, Gil-Sanchis C, Faus A, Ferro J, Pellicer A, et al. Identification and characterization of the human leiomyoma side population as putative tumor-initiating cells. Fertility and Sterility. 2012;**98**(3):741-751

[65] Tai CT, Lin WC, Chang WC, Chiu TH, Chen GT. Classical cadherin and catenin expression in normal myometrial tissues and uterine leiomyomas. Molecular Reproduction and Development: Incorporating Gamete Research. 2003;**64**(2):172-178

[66] Tanwar PS, Lee HJ, Zhang L, Zukerberg LR, Taketo MM, Rueda BR, et al. Constitutive activation of Beta-catenin in uterine stroma and smooth muscle leads to the development of mesenchymal tumors in mice. Biology of Reproduction. 2009;**81**(3):545-552

[67] Ono M, Yin P, Navarro A, Moravek MB, Coon JS, Druschitz SA, et al. Paracrine activation of WNT/β-catenin pathway in uterine leiomyoma stem cells promotes tumor growth. National Academy of Sciences of the United States of America. 2013;**110**(42):17053-17058

[68] Arici A, Sozen I. Transforming growth factor-β3 is expressed at high levels in leiomyoma where it stimulates fibronectin expression and cell proliferation. Fertility and Sterility. 2000;**73**(5):1006-1011

[69] Govindan S, Shaik NA, Vedicherla B, Kodati V, Rao KP, Hasan Q. Estrogen receptor-α gene (T/C) Pvu II polymorphism in endometriosis and uterine fibroids. Disease Markers. 2009;**26**(4):149-154

[70] Borahay MA, Al-Hendy A, Kilic GS, Boehning D. Signaling pathways in leiomyoma: Understanding pathobiology and implications for therapy. Molecular Medicine. 2015;**21**(1):242-256

[71] Levin ER. Plasma membrane estrogen receptors. Trends in Endocrinology & Metabolism. 2009;**20**(10):477-482

[72] Prossnitz ER, Arterburn JB, Smith HO, Oprea TI, Sklar LA, Hathaway HJ. Estrogen signaling through the transmembrane G protein-coupled receptor GPR30. Annual Review of Physiology. 2008;**70**(1):165-190

[73] Benassayag C, Leroy MJ, Rigourd V, Robert B, Honore JC, Mignot TM, et al. Estrogen receptors (ERα/ERβ) in normal and pathological growth of the human

myometrium: Pregnancy and leiomyoma. American Journal of Physiology-Endocrinology and Metabolism. 1999;**276**(6):E1112-E1118

[74] Jakimiuk AJ, Bogusiewicz M, Tarkowski R, Dziduch P, Adamiak A, Wróbel A, et al. Estrogen receptor α and β expression in uterine leiomyomas from premenopausal women. Fertility and Sterility. 2004;**82**:1244-1249

[75] Harris HR, Petrick JL, Rosenberg L. The epidemiology of uterine fibroids: Where do we go from here? Fertility and Sterility. 2022;**117**(4):841-842

[76] Ishikawa H, Reierstad S, Demura M, Rademaker AW, Kasai T, Inoue M, et al. High aromatase expression in uterine leiomyoma tissues of African-American women. The Journal of Clinical Endocrinology & Metabolism. 2009;**94**(5):1752-1756

[77] Imir AG, Lin Z, Yin P, Deb S, Yilmaz B, Cetin M, et al. Aromatase expression in uterine leiomyomata is regulated primarily by proximal promoters I. 3/II. The Journal of Clinical Endocrinology & Metabolism. 2007;**92**(5):1979-1982

[78] Ishikawa H, Fencki V, Marsh EE, Yin P, Chen D, Cheng YH, et al. CCAAT/enhancer binding protein β regulates aromatase expression via multiple and novel cis-regulatory sequences in uterine leiomyoma. The Journal of Clinical Endocrinology & Metabolism. 2008;**93**(3):981-991

[79] Parsanezhad ME, Azmoon M, Alborzi S, Rajaeefard A, Zarei A, Kazerooni T, et al. A randomized, controlled clinical trial comparing the effects of aromatase inhibitor (letrozole) and gonadotropin-releasing hormone agonist (triptorelin) on uterine leiomyoma volume and hormonal status. Fertility and Sterility. 2010;**93**(1):192-198

[80] Maruo T, Ohara N, Wang J, Matsuo H. Sex steroidal regulation of uterine leiomyoma growth and apoptosis. Human Reproduction Update. 2004;**10**(3):207-220

[81] Nierth-Simpson EN, Martin MM, Chiang TC, Melnik LI, Rhodes LV, Muir SE, et al. Human uterine smooth muscle and leiomyoma cells differ in their rapid 17β-estradiol signaling: Implications for proliferation. Endocrinology. 2009;**150**(5):2436-2445

[82] Toprani SM, Kelkar MV. Role of DNA damage and repair mechanisms in uterine fibroid/leiomyomas: A review. Biology of Reproduction. 2021;**104**(1):58-70

[83] Hassan MH, Salama SA, Arafa HM, Hamada FM, Al-Hendy A. Adenovirus-mediated delivery of a dominant-negative estrogen receptor gene in uterine leiomyoma cells abrogates estrogen-and progesterone-regulated gene expression. The Journal of Clinical Endocrinology & Metabolism. 2007;**92**(10):3949-3957

[84] Veronica M, Ali A, Venkateshwari A, Mamata D, Nallari P. Association of estrogen and progesterone receptor gene polymorphisms and their respective hormones in uterine leiomyomas. Tumor Biology. 2016;**37**(6):8067-8074

[85] Alali OM, Churnosov MI. The etiopathogenesis of uterine leiomyomas: A review. Gynecology. 2023;**25**(1):22-30

[86] Ali M, Bariani MV, Vafaei S, Omran MM, Yang Q, Madueke-Laveaux OS, et al. Prevention of uterine fibroids: Molecular mechanisms and potential clinical application. Journal of Endometriosis and

Uterine Disorders. 2023;**1**:1-6. DOI: 10.1016/j.jeud.2023.100018

[87] Tanioka S, Asano R, Wakabayashi R, Hayashi H, Shigeta H. Possible significance of degeneration and decreased expression of progesterone receptor in postmenopausal uterine leiomyoma. BMC Women's Health. 2022;**22**(1):346

[88] Khan N, Afaq F, Saleem M, Ahmad N, Mukhtar H. Targeting multiple signaling pathways by green tea polyphenol (−)-epigallocatechin-3-gallate. Cancer Research. 2006;**66**(5):2500-2505

[89] Hoekstra AV, Sefton EC, Berry E, Lu Z, Hardt J, Marsh E, et al. Progestins activate the AKT pathway in leiomyoma cells and promote survival. The Journal of Clinical Endocrinology & Metabolism. 2009;**94**(5):1768-1774

[90] Reis FM, Bloise E, Ortiga-Carvalho TM. Hormones and pathogenesis of uterine fibroids. Best Practice & Research Clinical Obstetrics & Gynaecology. 2016;**34**:13-24

[91] Yin P, Roqueiro D, Huang L, Owen JK, Xie A, Navarro A, et al. Genome-wide progesterone receptor binding: Cell type-specific and shared mechanisms in T47D breast cancer cells and primary leiomyoma cells. PLoS One. 2012;**7**(1):e29021

[92] Yin P, Lin Z, Reierstad S, Wu J, Ishikawa H, Marsh EE, et al. Transcription factor KLF11 integrates progesterone receptor signaling and proliferation in uterine leiomyoma cells KLF11 as a novel PR target gene. Cancer Research. 2010;**70**(4):1722-1730

[93] Segars JH, Parrott EC, Nagel JD, Guo XC, Gao X, Birnbaum LS, et al. Proceedings from the third National Institutes of Health international congress on advances in uterine leiomyoma research: Comprehensive review, conference summary and future recommendations. Human Reproduction Update. 2014;**20**(3):309-333

[94] Yu L, Moore AB, Dixon D. Receptor tyrosine kinases and their hormonal regulation in uterine leiomyoma. Seminars in Reproductive Medicine. 2010;**28**(03):250-259

[95] Ying Z, Weiyuan Z. Dual actions of progesterone on uterine leiomyoma correlate with the ratio of progesterone receptor a: B. Gynecological Endocrinology. 2009;**25**(8):520-523

[96] Donnez J, Vázquez F, Tomaszewski J, Nouri K, Bouchard P, Fauser BC, et al. Long-term treatment of uterine fibroids with ulipristal acetate☆. Fertility and Sterility. 2014;**101**(6):1565-1573

[97] Chung JE, Kurisawa M, Kim YJ, Uyama H, Kobayashi S. Amplification of antioxidant activity of catechin by polycondensation with acetaldehyde. Biomacromolecules. 2004;**5**(1):113-118

[98] Ahmed RS, Liu G, Renzetti A, Farshi P, Yang H, Soave C, et al. Biological and mechanistic characterization of novel prodrugs of green tea polyphenol epigallocatechin gallate analogs in human leiomyoma cell lines. Journal of Cellular Biochemistry. 2016;**117**(10):2357-2369

[99] Tsuiji K, Takeda T, Li B, Wakabayashi A, Kondo A, Kimura T, et al. Inhibitory effect of curcumin on uterine leiomyoma cell proliferation. Gynecological Endocrinology. 2011;**27**(7):512-517

[100] Halder SK, Goodwin JS, Al-Hendy A. 1, 25-Dihydroxyvitamin D3 reduces TGF-β3-induced fibrosis-related

gene expression in human uterine leiomyoma cells. The Journal of Clinical Endocrinology & Metabolism. 2011;**96**(4):E754-E762

[101] Lee TK, Kim DI, Song YL, Lee YC, Kim HM, Kim CH. Differential inhibition of Scutellaria barbata D. Don (Lamiaceae) on HCG-promoted proliferation of cultured uterine leiomyomal and myometrial smooth muscle cells. Immunopharmacology and Immunotoxicology. 2004;**26**(3):329-342

[102] Wu HL, Chuang TY, Al-Hendy A, Diamond MP, Azziz R, Chen YH. Berberine inhibits the proliferation of human uterine leiomyoma cells. Fertility and Sterility. 2015;**103**(4):1098-1106

[103] Salehi AM, Jenabi E, Farashi S, Aghababaei S, Salimi Z. The environmental risk factors related to uterine leiomyoma: An umbrella review. Journal of Gynecology Obstetrics and Human Reproduction. 2022;**52**:102517

[104] Ho Y, Yang YC, Chin YT, Chou SY, Chen YR, Shih YJ, et al. Resveratrol inhibits human leiomyoma cell proliferation via crosstalk between integrin αvβ3 and IGF-1R. Food and Chemical Toxicology. 2018;**120**:346-355

[105] Li L, Qiu RL, Lin Y, Cai Y, Bian Y, Fan Y, et al. Resveratrol suppresses human cervical carcinoma cell proliferation and elevates apoptosis via the mitochondrial and p53 signaling pathways. Oncology Letters. 2018;**15**(6):9845-9851

[106] Collins KG, Fitzgerald GF, Stanton C, Ross RP. Looking beyond the terrestrial: The potential of seaweed derived bioactives to treat non-communicable diseases. Marine Drugs. 2016;**14**(3):60

[107] Charboneau AJ, Delaney JP, Beilman G. Fucoidans inhibit the formation of post-operative abdominal adhesions in a rat model. PLoS One. 2018;**13**(11):e0207797

[108] Li X, Wu N, Chen Y, Tan J, Wang J, Geng L, et al. Degradation of different molecular weight fucoidans and their inhibition of TGF-β1 induced epithelial–mesenchymal transition in mouse renal tubular epithelial cells. International Journal of Biological Macromolecules. 2020;**151**:545-553

[109] Gajowik A, Dobrzyńska MM. The evaluation of protective effect of lycopene against genotoxic influence of X-irradiation in human blood lymphocytes. Radiation and Environmental Biophysics. 2017;**56**(4):413-422

[110] Rao AV, Rao LG. Carotenoids and human health. Pharmacological Research. 2007;**55**(3):207-216

[111] Khan N, Mukhtar H. Tea polyphenols for health promotion. Life Sciences. 2007;**81**(7):519-533

[112] Corachán A, Ferrero H, Escrig J, Monleon J, Faus A, Cervelló I, et al. Long-term vitamin D treatment decreases human uterine leiomyoma size in a xenograft animal model. Fertility and Sterility. 2020;**113**(1):205-216

[113] Ciebiera M, Męczekalski B, Łukaszuk K, Jakiel G. Potential synergism between ulipristal acetate and vitamin D3 in uterine fibroid pharmacotherapy–2 case studies. Gynecological Endocrinology. 2019;**35**(6):473-477

[114] Wang Y, Feng G, Wang J, Zhou Y, Liu Y, Shi Y, et al. Differential effects of tumor necrosis factor-α on matrix metalloproteinase-2 expression

in human myometrial and uterine leiomyoma smooth muscle cells. Human Reproduction. 2015;**30**(1):61-70

[115] Wu XJ, Guo Q, Cao BS, Tan LX, Zhang HY, Cai YR, et al. Uterine leiomyomas: Safety and efficacy of US-guided suprapubic transvaginal radiofrequency ablation at 1-year follow-up. Radiology. 2016;**279**(3):952-960

[116] Wang LU, Zhang P, Li X, Zhang YI, Zhan Q, Wang C. Low-molecular-weight fucoidan attenuates bleomycin-induced pulmonary fibrosis: Possible role in inhibiting TGF-β1-induced epithelial-mesenchymal transition through ERK pathway. American Journal of Translational Research. 2019;**11**(4):2590

[117] Chen HY, Huang TC, Lin LC, Shieh TM, Wu CH, Wang KL, et al. Fucoidan inhibits the proliferation of leiomyoma cells and decreases extracellular matrix-associated protein expression. Cellular Physiology and Biochemistry. 2018;**49**(5):1970-1986

[118] Cho KS, Shin M, Kim S, Lee SB. Recent advances in studies on the therapeutic potential of dietary carotenoids in neurodegenerative diseases. Oxidative Medicine and Cellular Longevity. 2018;**2018**:1-13